Colin A. Espie PhD, DSc(Med) is Professor of Sleep Medicine in the Nuffield Department of Clinical Neurosciences and a Fellow of Somerville College, University of Oxford. He is Director of the Experimental and Clinical Sleep Medicine programme within the Sleep and Circadian Neuroscience Institute, and Clinical Director of the Oxford Online Programme in Sleep Medicine. Dr Espie has authored/co-authored over three hundred publications and books, particularly on CBT, and is co-founder of Big Health (Sleepio) which develops digital interventions for insomnia.

The aim of the **Overcoming** series is to enable people with a range of common problems and disorders to take control of their own recovery programme.

Each title, with its specially tailored programme, is devised by a practising clinician using the latest techniques of cognitive behavioural therapy – techniques which have been shown to be highly effective in changing the way patients think about themselves and their problems.

Many books in the Overcoming series are recommended under the Reading Well scheme.

OVERCOMING INSOMNIA

2nd Edition

A self-help guide using cognitive behavioural techniques

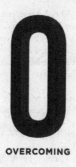

OVERCOMING

COLIN A. ESPIE

ROBINSON

ROBINSON

First published in Great Britain in 2006 by Robinson,
an imprint of Constable & Robinson Ltd

This revised and updated edition published by Robinson in 2021

3 5 7 9 10 8 6 4 2

IMPORTANT NOTE
This book is not intended as a substitute for medical advice or treatment.
Any person with a condition requiring medical attention should consult a
qualified medical practitioner or suitable therapist.

A CIP catalogue record for this book
is available from the British Library.

ISBN: 978-1-47214-141-5

Typeset in Bembo by Initial Typesetting Services, Edinburgh

Printed in Italy by Elcograf S.p.A.

Papers used by Robinson are from well-managed forests
and other responsible sources.

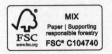

Robinson
An imprint of
Little, Brown Book Group
Carmelite House
50 Victoria Embankment
London EC4Y 0DZ

The authorised representative
in the EEA is
Hachette Ireland
8 Castlecourt Centre
Dublin 15, D15 XTP3, Ireland
(email: info@hbgi.ie)

An Hachette UK Company
www.hachette.co.uk

www.littlebrown.co.uk

To Aud: my wife and my soulmate

Contents

Part One:
Understanding Insomnia

Part Two:
Assessing Your Sleep and
Your Insomnia

Part Three:
Overcoming Your Insomnia
and Becoming a Good Sleeper

Part Four:
Special Circumstances

Acknowledgements

I would like to thank a number of people who have made a major contribution, in various ways, to the work underlying this book. They are too many to mention by name, but I hope that by summarising I can adequately reflect my very sincere gratitude.

First of all, I am grateful to the many colleagues I have known and worked with over the years across Europe, the USA, Canada, Australia, Asia and, of course, in the UK. The development and evaluation of CBT for insomnia has been, and continues to be, an international effort, and I have been privileged to be part of that work.

Then there is my own team at the University of Oxford in the Sleep and Circadian Neuroscience Institute (SCNi). I particularly want to thank my colleagues in the SCNi's Experimental and Clinical Sleep Medicine group, and also those who worked with me previously when I was Director of University of Glasgow Sleep Centre. Scores of highly motivated clinicians, research fellows, research assistants, technologists, postgraduates and administrative staff have helped to keep the show on the road! More than that – these people have been the lifeblood of my professional life.

I also want to thank my colleagues and the staff at Big Health (https://www.bighealth.com/) where, since 2008, we have been working on developing, testing and clinically validating *Sleepio*™, a digital CBT programme that delivers effective help in overcoming insomnia on the web and on mobile devices.

None of this, of course, would have been possible without our patients and research participants, from whom we find out, through one research method or another, everything that we know about the perplexing yet intriguing disorder that we call 'insomnia'.

Finally, I have a wonderful and supportive family of whom I am immensely proud . . . Craig who is fulfilling his father's alternative dream by playing music professionally (https://skerryvore.com/), Carolyn who is following in our footsteps through her practice as a Clinical Psychologist in the NHS in Scotland, and our youngest, Robbie, who is now in his final year of study at the University of Edinburgh Law School. We are also doting grandparents of Mia, Ella, Callum and Charlie – four more reasons to be immensely proud and happy. Most of all, there is my alluring and very special wife, Audrey, to whom I dedicate this book with all my love.

Preface

The priorities and pressures are such that most of us in academic life spend the majority of our time conducting research, analysing data, writing scientific papers, teaching our students and training health professionals for practice. Those of us who are clinical academics also try to fit in seeing the occasional patient or two! In this context, writing books for the general public is at best regarded as a hobby; at worst even a misuse of our time! Yet what is the purpose of knowledge if it is not to share it, and to try to improve things for people?

I struggled with this dilemma for a while. However, I decided in 2006, after being approached by the publishers, that the time had finally come to 'do the self-help book'! I am sure that other authors in the excellent CBT series that Little, Brown produce have probably felt the same way. I guess most of us have a lay readership book in us! Well for better or for worse . . . this one is mine. I have now got round to writing this long overdue 2ⁿᵈ edition. My apologies to the team at Little, Brown for being rather elusive; but thank you so much for your support in putting this revised edition together.

Re-writing the book has given me the opportunity to make available to you the treatment materials that we have developed and evaluated in our research studies. I have tried as best as I can, within the confines of the written word, also to make those elements of treatment personalised to you. What you are getting here is pretty much a complete CBT treatment guide for insomnia; the way I would present it to you if you came to my clinic in Oxford. I make no apology for excluding the many other supposed 'sleep solutions' that are promoted to the public as new and life-changing – except that there is no trustworthy evidence for them. I am sure that you will agree that sleep matters, and that insomnia is an important health problem. So, I will only be telling you about evidence-based approaches that meet the highest standards of scientific and clinical scrutiny. That is the principal reason that I am confident that you have a very powerful tool in your hands that will help you towards overcoming your insomnia.

Forms and questionnaires printed in the book, together with other useful resources, are now also available online at https://www.colinespie.com.

I wish you success as you set out on this 'course' of CBT treatment . . . sleep soundly and sleep well!

Colin A. Espie
BSc, MAppSci, PhD, DSc(Med),
CPsychol, CSci. FBPsS, FRSM, FAASM
University of Oxford
August 2021

General Introduction

To be unable to sleep is one of life's worst experiences! Insomnia affects not only the night-time, through disrupted and unsatisfactory sleep, but it also has consequences in terms of daytime symptoms and quality of life. People with persistent sleep problems often complain of being mentally slowed and irritable or moody during the day. What is more, they are not the only ones to suffer! Broken sleep can affect partners, children, and our social life and working life.

Insomnia is a major public health problem. Billions of dollars are spent worldwide every year on prescribed medications, over-the-counter remedies, and other suggested solutions – all in the search for a decent sleep. One in ten adults, and one in five of those over 65 years of age have insomnia. Being unable to sleep is one of the most common complaints heard by primary care practitioners, yet our healthcare systems are barely scratching the surface in offering a service that will help people.

Research conducted over the past 40 years has established Cognitive Behavioural Therapy (CBT) as an effective treatment for persistent insomnia. Indeed, leading authorities now regard CBT as the treatment of first choice. Let me just say that again, CBT is the intervention that is recommended for chronic insomnia in clinical guidelines throughout the world. Not sleeping pills (of any kind), yet that is just about all that people get offered. Why? Well, there is a problem – CBT is not widely available; in some places it is hardly available at all. Clinical Psychology, Psychological Therapy, and Behavioural Medicine services do not have the capacity to meet the potential demand. Besides, they spend most of their time on the (also) very common problems of depression, anxiety and other mental health disorders. Yet the research has been conducted on insomnia, the evidence is there, but the means to deliver CBT is so far still lagging behind. I hope that this book goes some way to filling that gap for you.

As one of the people who has been most closely involved with the development and evaluation of insomnia treatment, I want to help you to sleep well. I believe that one of the ways to help overcome the scale of the insomnia problem that is out there is to put the solution, the CBT itself, directly into your hands. Hence this book, and digital CBT solutions like Sleepio™. We as professionals must, and will, continue to lobby politicians and healthcare providers to develop much needed services. However, there is also a lot that you can do to improve your sleep yourself, if you are given the right tools for the job.

This book is designed for your use as a complete course of CBT treatment. I have set out the different parts of the book, and the chapters within each part, so that you can use it as a CBT programme. You are about to set out on a course of therapy. I will be your therapist, as it were, from a distance, but you must take on the role not only of patient but also of collaborator and co-therapist. You will be learning and implementing at the same time . . . you will be evaluating progress . . . you will get what you give! Like any course of treatment, I ask you to take this CBT programme seriously. Give it some of your best quality time and attention. Your sleep is worth it.

The Return of the Dove

Early in my career, I guess it was in the mid 1980s, I was inspired by the writing of Viktor Frankl (1905–1997) who, just after World War II, published a book titled *Man's Search for Meaning*, based on his experiences surviving several Nazi death camps. Frankl went on to become a leading Austrian neurologist and psychiatrist; but instinctively he was a remarkable philosopher and psychologist. A turn of phrase in another of his books that was written around the same time caught my eye – and caught my imagination. It still does. In *The Doctor and the Soul*, Frankl recalls this statement from the famous Swiss psychiatrist Paul Dubois (1848–1918):

> *Sleep is like a dove which has landed near one's hand and stays there as long as one does not pay any attention to it. But if one attempts to grab it, it quickly flies away.*

Here Dubois captures the essence of sleep, and also of the dilemma facing the person with insomnia. In the good times, sleep just sits there alongside us, largely unnoticed. Sleep, like the dove, just becomes part of the natural environment. It's comfortable with us and we are comfortable with it. The dove remains at peace in the world of the good sleeper, because the good sleeper really doesn't think about it. The good sleeper doesn't know how to sleep. It just happens. There's really no need to pay too much attention to it.

Contrast this with the person with insomnia. When you so much want and need sleep it's very hard not to become pre-occupied with it. You crave it, you want it to come, you are looking out for it, you try to find ways to attract it to you. When it comes, you hope it will stay, you worry that it will not, and so often it has not stayed. So, you become like the person paying too much attention to the dove, trying lovingly to grab hold of it . . . and it quickly flies away.

Does this sound familiar?

CBT offers you the prospect of the return of the dove. Join me in helping you to bring sleep back. A sleep that will stay. The cognitive and behavioural techniques that you will learn directly address all those things that get in the way of sleep. So now let's start . . . let's overcome insomnia together . . . let's get back to normal good sleep!

PART ONE

UNDERSTANDING INSOMNIA

Introduction to Part One

The first part of the book is about developing an understanding of sleep and an understanding of insomnia. I hope you will find that this is a helpful step towards your goal, of learning how to overcome insomnia and learning how to become a good sleeper.

In the 1st edition I said, *'Try not to be tempted to jump ahead to Part Two, especially if you are the kind of person who likes to "get on with it"! Part One will give you important background information that will make it much easier to put into practice your cognitive behavioural treatment.'* This is true.

But you know what, I've changed my mind about being so prescriptive; because it is entirely up to you! To be clear, I'm not saying now that it's a bad idea to read Part One first; but another possibility is to read it in parallel. If you want to do that, it's perfectly fine too. I realise that you might be ready right now to start to work on your sleep problems, and I want to make sure that I'm the last person to prevent that!

Introduction to Part One

1

Understanding Normal Sleep

What is Sleep?

You may be surprised by this, but I would like to begin by explaining what sleep is not! This is important because sleep is very commonly misunderstood.

First, sleep is *not* simply the absence of wakefulness. Falling asleep is not like having your light-switch in the 'off' position, compared with wakefulness being like a light that is switched 'on'. The on/off idea would suggest that we live our lives either at one extreme or the other. This is not in fact correct because there is variation within sleep, just as there is variation within wakefulness. You are not always 'wide awake' . . . are you? Similarly, you are not always 'fast asleep'. We can also be awake and asleep at the same time. I can sense your surprise right now. Are you intrigued? Well, more on that to come.

Second, sleep is *not* an inactive process. Sleep is not 'down tools' time, or a kind of respite or escape. On the contrary, the very activities of sleep are absolutely vital to life. Your sleep is a part of your life, not something separate from it – you will have heard it said that we spend one-third of our lives asleep (I hear you say, 'I wish!'). Just because we are unconscious and have no memory for the greater part of our sleep, does not mean that sleep is either a simple or a passive state.

So, what then *is* sleep? The famous Israeli scientist Dr Peretz Lavie once wrote a semi-autobiographical book about his experiences in sleep research. He called the book *The Enchanted World of Sleep*. For me this title captures the fact that sleep is rich and diverse and precious; and still fascinatingly mysterious. We live our lives not just in the waking world. Let's go and take a glimpse at life within sleep.

Research studies have shown us that sleep is a very complex, yet a very ordered process. Scientists have discovered the complexity of sleep by studying the activity of the brain during overnight sleep laboratory recordings. Sleep is made up of different subtypes and stages. Sleep is also orderly because these types and stages of sleep are organised in a series of cycles that repeat across the night. You can see then that sleep is an active process in terms of brain activity. However, it is also active in other ways. For example, it is during sleep that our body tissue is repaired. Proteins, the building blocks of life, are manufactured during sleep and some hormones are produced selectively during the night, like growth hormone in developing infants and children. So, there is some truth in the idea that we grow during the night! These are just examples of physical processes during sleep, but there are also very important mental processes. We catch a glimpse of this in the phenomenon of dreaming. Of course, we do not always wake out of our dreams, but when we do what is very apparent is that we have been thinking, even though we were asleep. Enchanting!

The section coming up is quite technical. I think you will find it interesting, so please do read on! However, if I lose you at times, don't worry. The take-home message is that although sleep is complex, with many different stages and phases, it is wonderfully coordinated so that each element of sleep plays an important role throughout our lives in preparing us for the day ahead and in keeping us physically and mentally healthy.

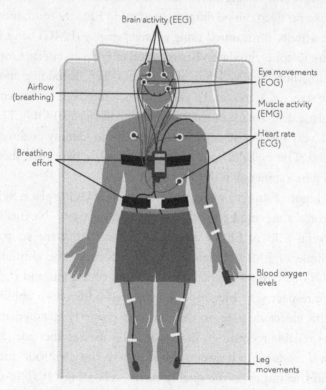

Figure 1: Sleep lab assessment

Measuring sleep in the laboratory

In order to understand this complex process, it may be helpful to find out a little about the objective assessment of sleep, and this is usually done in a *sleep laboratory*.

Scientists and clinicians study sleep by taking three types of measurement. First, electrical activity in the brain is measured by *electroencephalography* (EEG). This measure is used because the EEG signals associated with wakefulness are different from those found during sleep. Also, the different *sleep stages* that make up sleep can be differentiated using EEG. Second, muscle activity is measured using *electromyography* (EMG) because muscle 'tone' also differs between wakefulness and sleep. Once again, there are EMG differences within sleep, depending upon the stage of sleep that the person is in. Third, eye movements during sleep are measured using *electro-oculography* (EOG). This is a very specific measurement that helps to identify dreaming sleep. The eyeballs make characteristic movements that show us when someone is in this type of sleep.

Figure 1 shows a typical sleep assessment taking place. Skin *electrodes* are used to pick up electrical activity. Normally, several pairs of EEG electrodes are attached to the scalp, a couple of EMG electrodes are placed under the chin and EOG electrodes are placed at the side of the left and right eye respectively. Electrodes may be self-adhesive or applied with electrode glue, so that they are properly attached and get reliable recordings. Electrode gel is used to increase *electrical conductivity* between the skin and the electrode itself and this improves the quality of the recordings. It all looks a bit uncomfortable, but it does tell us a lot about sleep!

So, what would happen if we looked at normal sleep in a laboratory using EEG, EMG and EOG?

Wakefulness

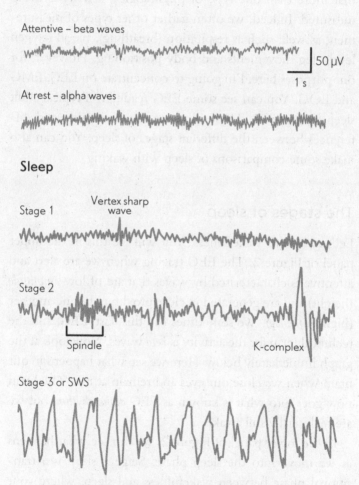

Attentive – beta waves

50 μV

1 s

At rest – alpha waves

Sleep

Stage 1

Vertex sharp wave

Stage 2

Spindle

K-complex

Stage 3 or SWS

Figure 2: A polysomnographic (PSG) recording
showing the different stages of NREM sleep

This whole system of assessment is called *polysomnography* (PSG) as a shorthand way of describing a full sleep assessment – the prefix 'poly' simply referring to the fact that more than one type of physiological activity is being measured. Indeed, we often gather other types of measurement as well; such as respiration (breathing), blood oxygen levels, leg movements and body positioning. However, for our purposes here, I'm going to concentrate on EEG, EMG and EOG. You can see some EEG readings of typical adult sleep in Figure 2. These illustrate the similarities and differences between the different stages of sleep. You can also make some comparisons of sleep with waking.

The stages of sleep

Let's start with wakefulness. You will see this in the upper panel of Figure 2. The EEG tracing when we are alert and attentive is characterised by waves that are of low *amplitude* (height) and are generated in close proximity to one another (high *frequency*). We sometimes call this 'fast' EEG, and the technical term for the activity is *beta* waves. Now look at the graph immediately below. Here we see what happens in our brain when we close our eyes and remain at rest. The brain now goes into what is known as EEG *alpha rhythm*, but we are technically still awake.

In the lower panel of Figure 2, we can see what happens as we move into the sleep phase. Stage 1 sleep is a transitional phase between wakefulness and sleep, where your EEG waves slow down to around 3 to 7 *cycles per second* (cps). These are known as *theta* waves. You may actually be aware of 'dropping off' or someone may observe that you are. Your muscles begin to lose their EMG *tone* (that is they relax) in comparison with wakefulness. Similarly, if we were monitoring your EOG, the traces would begin to show *slow rolling eye movements*. Stage 1 sleep normally lasts only a matter of minutes of drowsiness before progressing into the second stage of sleep.

If you look at stage 2 sleep on the lower panel of Figure 2, you will see that the EEG varies quite considerably. These are what we call *mixed frequency* EEG waves (some fast, some slow, some high amplitude, some low). However, there are two characteristic formations that occur repeatedly, and these are the defining features of stage 2 sleep. The *K-complex* takes it names from the shape of an initially descending and then ascending sharp change in voltage. If you are trying to make sense of this by following Figure 2, you will need to know that by tradition upward deflections of EEG are 'descending' and downward deflections are 'ascending' – just to confuse you! The other features of stage 2 sleep are known as *sleep spindles*. This is a descriptive term for rapid bursts of high frequency EEG activity (12–14 cps) that occur intermittently, sometimes just after a K-complex. Although stage 2 comprises the largest proportion of adult sleep (50–60 per cent), the very first phase of the night's stage 2 sleep is usually quite short.

We have the deepest part of our sleep during the first couple of hours of the night and there is a rapid transition into this stage 3 sleep during this period. It seems like the brain wants to get us into this *slow wave sleep* as quickly as possible. If you look at stage 3 sleep in Figure 2, you will see that the EEG trace now reveals higher amplitude waves occurring at much lower frequency. In other words, the waves have slowed down, they are high rollers. We call them *delta* waves. Their amplitude will be 75 *microvolts* (μV) or greater and the wave frequency has now dropped to its lowest at ½–2 cps. Deep sleep is a form of *synchronised sleep* because the brain's electrical activity settles to a harmonised rhythm and produces the steady 'beats' that you can see in Figure 2. I'm sure you must be thinking that deep sleep like this sounds just the kind of sleep you would want. However, stage 3 only occupies up to 15–20 per cent of the night; and this should remind us that all stages of sleep are needed for a balanced sleep diet!

So far then, we can see the transition from wakefulness through to stage 3 sleep involves not only a loss of consciousness, but also a steady change in the EEG wave pattern from fast to slow activity, and that several stages of sleep can be differentiated. However, in 1953 two researchers in Chicago, Dr Nathaniel Kleitman, and his assistant Dr Eugene Aserinsky, made a crucial discovery about sleep. They noticed that there was another form of sleep during which the eyeballs moved rapidly, whereas the rest of the body was pretty much paralysed. The term *rapid eye movement sleep (REM sleep)* was coined, and so important was its discovery that the previously described stages 1, 2 and 3 of sleep actually became known as non-rapid eye movement sleep, or for short, *non-REM* or *NREM sleep*!

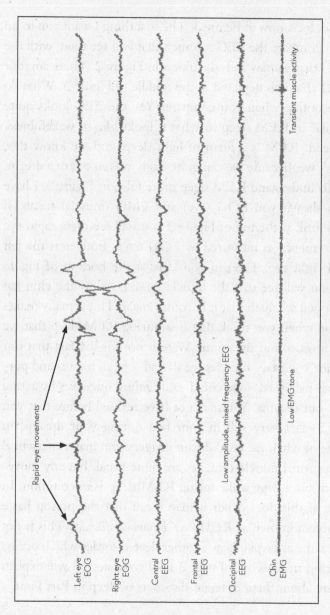

Figure 3: PSG recording showing REM sleep

So, look now at Figure 3. The first thing I want you to do is to compare the EEG channels that you see there with the EEG that we saw in wakefulness in Figure 2. There are four EEG channels depicted in the middle of Figure 3. What do you notice when you compare? Yes, the EEG looks quite similar in REM sleep to what it looks like in wakefulness. Indeed, REM is a form of light sleep, and we know this, don't we, because we can quite easily waken out of a dream.

To understand REM sleep more fully, in Figure 3, I have also shown you EOG (eye) and EMG (muscle) traces. If you look at the top of Figure 3 you will see these rapid eye movements, as measured by EOG traces from near the left and right eye. Then, if you look at the bottom of Figure 3, you will see that the muscle tension below the chin has dropped so much that it becomes *atonic*. This actually makes sense when you think that it is during REM sleep that we do most of our dreaming. Were it not for the fact that our major voluntary muscles are flaccid – to all intents and purposes paralysed – we could easily injure ourselves by acting out our dreams. You may not have realised before that you are in fact very still in your bed during your dreams, in spite of whatever vivid dream imagery you may experience! Occasional muscle twitches are quite usual, but any movement on a large scale during REM sleep is uncommon. In fact, if this does occur it may mean that the person has a problem known as *REM sleep behaviour disorder*. This is not the same as *sleepwalking*, another sleep disorder which occurs during arousals out of stage 3 slow wave sleep. I will explain more about these different disorders of sleep in Part Four.

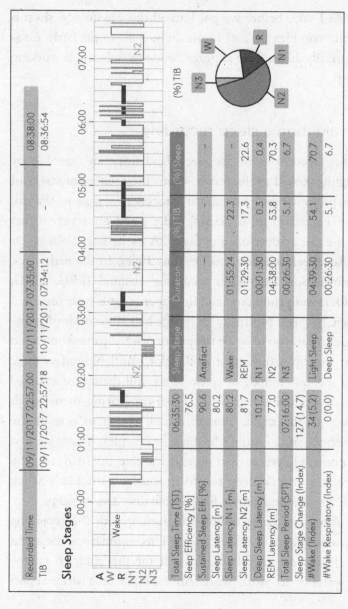

Figure 4: Sleep report

As I said, before we got into all this physiology, sleep is quite complex isn't it? Fortunately, it all works fairly automatically, like a dove at peace beside us, when it is working well.

Evaluating a sleep recording

Sleep records from the sleep laboratory are *scored* – by highly trained professionals – into these different stages of sleep. Sometimes we call this process *staging sleep*. We still use a standard set of scoring rules based on a system that was expertly developed in the USA in the late 1960s by Dr Allan Rechtschaffen and Dr Tony Kales. In the early days, information from each recording channel (EEG, EMG, EOG) was printed out and the paper records were reviewed page by page. Normally each page had 30 seconds of print-out, so can you imagine the pile of printed paper you would get from just one night in the sleep lab?! Nowadays these 30 second chunks, or *epochs* as we call them, are analysed on a monitor screen and the person scoring them scrolls through the night, allocating each epoch to one of the sleep stages, according to the scoring rules. There are also automated sleep analysis systems available, but many labs still prefer to check sleep records manually, particularly when we are assessing people for possible disorders of sleep.

After a sleep recording has been scored, the recording system generates a *sleep report*. This summarises the night and provides useful information for the clinician or the researcher to work with. An example of a sleep report from my own lab can be seen in Figure 4. Let me take you through the information presented there.

This sleep report is on a healthy 25-year-old female, and I am using it simply to illustrate sleep scoring. As you can see, at the top of Figure 4, the recording started just prior to 11 p.m. and ended around 7:30 a.m., with a total time in bed (TIB) of 8 hours 36 minutes.

Looking next at the complex graph of sleep stages, from left to right we have time on the x-axis; and from top to bottom on the y-axis we have the sleep stages themselves.

From visual inspection, we see that she was awake for quite a while, first falling into NREM stage 1 sleep (N1) around 00:20hr; but transitioning rapidly into NREM stage 2 (N2) and then NREM stage 3 (N3). This first *cycle* of NREM sleep ended with a few wake spells occurring between 01:00hr and 01:30hr. Then there was another small burst of stage 3 slow wave sleep prior to the first REM sleep period. This occurred about 70 minutes after falling asleep.

Looking then at around the 02:00hr time point, you can see that our subject is in another cycle of NREM sleep (comprising mainly stage 2 with some stage 3), she has a few brief awakenings before cycling again into REM at around 03:00hr and then back into NREM until after 04:00hr. You will notice that stage 3 sleep is over for the night – indeed, it didn't occur beyond 02:40 – and that the sleep that she gets in the second half of the night is mainly NREM stage 2 and REM sleep.

You will also see that there are quite a few awakenings towards morning, as sleep gets lighter, and that the REM episodes are longer in duration as the night goes on. Altogether she has four cycles of REM sleep, with the final episode ending around 06:30hr. She finally wakens around 07:20hr.

Well done, you have navigated quite a complex chart . . . but what does it mean? The main thing I want to get across is that this *sleep architecture* (we call it a *hypnogram*) is fairly normal. It illustrates the cycles of sleep and the flow in and out of NREM and REM sleep. The overall percentages of sleep are also quite typical for a young person. The pie chart shows us that sleep stage 1 was proportionately very small, that stage 2 made up more than 60 per cent of the night, that stage 3 was only about 7 per cent of overall sleep, and that REM was approaching a quarter of the sleep period at 23 per cent. Sometimes in a sleep lab people get a bit less deep sleep/slow wave sleep than they would at home, but it is not uncommon to find stage 3 is small in proportion to the night. I might have expected 10–20 per cent (maximum).

You might also have noticed of course that our subject seemed to take a while to get to sleep and that she woke up (W) a fair bit. If we look then at the table of information in Figure 4, we can see that her total sleep time was 6 hours 35 minutes because she took 80 minutes to fall asleep (sleep latency) and she was awake for a total of 1 hour 55 minutes. This gave her a sleep efficiency of 76 per cent, meaning that she was awake for 25 per cent of the time she spent in bed. This young woman then appears to have difficulties both getting to sleep and staying asleep. I guess we would call that insomnia.

Before leaving this topic, I want to take a moment more to consider whether or not people sleep normally in a sleep laboratory. You might be thinking that with all this equipment attached, your sleep continuity and sleep quality might be quite different . . . plus being in a strange environment! Quite so. A number of important studies investigating home versus lab-based PSG suggest that if PSG can be conducted at home it might be preferable. This is because people with insomnia associate their insomnia with their own bedroom environment. In a lab, they might actually sleep better than usual, and not worse than usual. In part, this could be due simply to the change of environment. But another possibility is that they might not *expect* to be able to sleep in a lab, and those lower expectations could mean that they will be less anxious about sleep and so sleep better. This research work then also introduces us to one of the psychological components to insomnia – the importance of expectations. In Oxford, we conduct both in-lab and home recordings, depending on the circumstances. It is good that technology has moved on to such an extent that it is quite feasible to get reliable, good quality PSG measurement using lightweight equipment that is suitable for home use.

What about personal devices that measure sleep?

People often come to the clinic saying that they have been *tracking* their sleep for some time. Usually they do this by means of a *wearable device*, such as a watch or other wrist or body monitor; or some form of headband. However, other devices that are not wearable are also becoming common.

These are typically *environmental sensors* placed in the bed (e.g. under the mattress, huggable pillows) or as fashionable objects positioned close to the bed.

All these personal devices attempt to estimate sleep and wakefulness using physiological information or motor activity, and many devices use data from more than one source. Examples include body movement, sleeping position, heart or pulse rate, breathing rate, oxygen levels in the bloodstream, skin conductance and EEG activity. Environmental sensors are often designed to pick up information on things that are thought to influence sleep, e.g. temperature (in the bed, in the bedroom), humidity, air quality, noise, light levels and, of course, time. Data are gathered so that a computerised element of the wearable or environmental device can use *algorithms* to feed back to you a representation of how you slept, and also to suggest what you should do to improve your sleep. In this way you can also track whether or not the steps you take make a difference to your sleep.

There are many devices of these types now available on the market, and they are becoming more sophisticated, more attractive and typically less expensive as time goes on. Indeed, sleep is often expected now as a 'feature' on wearable devices, amongst many other features to track exercise, diet and general health.

The key thing is – do they help?

Well, there are definitely two good things about them. First, using a device suggests that you are interested in self-care and in developing a healthier lifestyle; and second, that you may wish to explore sleep as part of that, and to make improvements to your sleep pattern. For example, some people may want to try to get more sleep if their lifestyle is poor.

All this seems reasonable, perhaps; so, what's the harm? Well, in the good sleeper, the potential for good most probably outweighs the potential for harm. The wearable device helps you stick to a better sleep habit and routine, and the feedback from the device (likely) indicates that you are a good sleeper. However, even in these circumstances, data from wearables can cause alarm. What if you think you slept rather well, and the device suggests it was a poor sleep last night? What are you to think? What are you to believe? What are you to do?

I've heard people say that, *'I thought I was a good sleeper until I started wearing a [device]; now I worry that my sleep isn't what it should be'*. In extreme cases, some people can develop an obsessive concern about their sleep, checking immediately upon waking up how they have slept, and becoming preoccupied with controlling sleep and making it better and better. Indeed, in the clinical and scientific literature the term *orthosomnia* is now being used to describe this new sleep problem that is largely caused by the availability and marketing of devices.

People also ask me, *'should I be concerned about my sleep . . . I'm only getting 25 per cent of my night in deep sleep'*. They assume that deep sleep is what your sleep ought to be, and that more and more deep sleep must surely be a good and necessary thing. However, you see, depending on your age and stage in life, 25 per cent is actually rather a lot of slow wave sleep! As we have seen, even 10–20 per cent slow wave sleep in a healthy young person is quite normal; and in later life 5 per cent would be pretty good. This is an example of potential harm because using a device could actually increase anxiety and worry about sleep in someone who is a perfectly good sleeper . . . and, as we know, worry about sleep is a contributory factor to the development and maintenance of insomnia.

All this said, I am reasonably confident that most good sleepers will have no problem with a wearable, and that many people will think they are great, will have a good experience, and will say that they have helped.

My greater concern is for people who have a sleep problem. Here the use of the device is not just out of curiosity, it is less likely to be simply a lifestyle companion. If you have insomnia and are concerned about it, there is an elevated risk that you could come to depend on the device and upon the data and advice it reports to you. At which point we need to ask the questions, are the data valid and reliable; and do the data help or hinder?

Wearables and environmental devices are not medical grade and they are not research grade instruments. This means that they don't have to pass rigorous tests concerning their performance or effectiveness. I'm not saying that they are unsafe, but I am questioning their usefulness for people who have a clinical problem with their sleep.

It needs to be recognised that people with chronic insomnia may be particularly vulnerable to the information that the device offers up. There is, I believe, a duty of care on the companies developing devices, therefore, to test directly, in large populations of people with insomnia, the validity of the sleep algorithms that lead to their sleep reports and to sleep advice.

From what I have seen so far, manufacturers of personal devices that are sold direct to the consumer have published trivial amounts of research on the performance of their devices in insomnia populations. Those data that have been published appear to be on samples of healthy, good sleepers. One cannot help but be concerned that the research that is available is not really there to support science or scientific discovery or to support sleep improvement in those who most need it, but to satisfy marketing claims. Granted, the devices will state that they are not intended for medical purposes. My point is that in the real world, people with established insomnia problems may be looking at spurious data. If the data from these personal devices is taken with a dose of scepticism, then there is less concern.

I also raised the question as to whether the data in any case help or hinder, even if the data are valid. This is more a point of principle about sleep data itself. I don't actually think much good purpose is served by 'knowing' how much objective sleep you got last night, or the composition of your sleep in terms of stages or phases, or what sleep stage you woke out of this morning. Over the course of my so far 40 years of experience as a clinician in the sleep field, and of conducting research on insomnia, there has never been a positive indication for quantifying sleep using PSG in the care of people with insomnia. Far less would there be an indication for routine PSG screening or evaluation of the wider population of good sleepers.

We absolutely do not need to know the architecture of our sleep. It isn't useful. It is a level of self-analysis that has no foundation in healthcare; and would likely cause confusion and anxiety. What devices are often trying to emulate is a laboratory style analysis of your sleep but taken in the comfort of your own home. But why? Even if you had insomnia, we wouldn't do this anywhere in the clinical world. Besides, these broad parameters of objective sleep, even supposing the device did measure them in a valid and reliable way, are largely irrelevant to the complaint of insomnia and to the treatment of insomnia. The subjective experience of sleep is simply not highly correlated to objective measures and good sleepers don't sleep well because they study their sleep.

All this said, I am sure that this section of the book will be amongst the parts that needs to be most frequently revised, and I will endeavour to keep things updated on social media! The technology is there, or nearly there, to measure the physiological and behavioural parameters of sleep accurately, and to close the existing gap between the wearable market and the medical device market. It remains to be seen who if anyone within the wearable technology industry will be willing to take the 'publish or perish' route, and who can solve the central challenge . . . which is about finding the best proxy for sleep complaint.

On the experience of sleep

You have perhaps used a wearable device, but probably never been to a sleep laboratory. In any event, I am sure you have tried to measure your sleep somehow! Perhaps by working out how long you think you have slept, or how long it took you to fall asleep, or how many times you woke up. These are measures of the *experience of sleep*, of what you remember about your sleep, and of the conclusions that you draw about your sleep. I bet you have found that it is not easy to calculate these things very accurately either!

You may even have tried to keep some type of *sleep diary* so that you can see what your sleep is like over a period of time, or to try to work out if there is a pattern. Diaries like this are very useful and we will be using them quite a bit as we assess and treat your insomnia. What I am saying is that your experience of sleep is very important, because that is what you have been living with.

Sometimes it is easier to think about the quality of our sleep, rather than its quantity. *Sleep quality* and sleep efficiency (which we will be thinking about quite a bit as we go on) have something in common. For example, you might feel that you have had a 'good sleep', or a 'deep sleep'; or perhaps more likely, that you have had a 'restless sleep' or 'hardly any sleep' or that it took you a 'long time to get into a proper sleep'. It is not always easy to convert these kinds of experience into numbers. Whether we are trying to estimate quantity or commenting on sleep quality, this is called *subjective assessment*. But we should not fall into the trap of thinking that subjective assessment is less important than objective assessment (such as PSG). What we think and feel about our sleep is terribly important, not least because it is our experience of sleep that relates most closely to the complaint of insomnia. This is usually what triggers help-seeking in the first place. Think of problems like depression or anxiety disorder as parallels. There is no objective test for either of these. They are subjective experiences and are treated on the basis of that subjective complaint. CBT works at this level.

It is likely that it was your experience of poor sleep that led you to be interested in this book in the first place. So, it will be important for you to keep accurate records of your subjective sleep experiences, and I will help you to make best use of a sleep diary. This is the form of assessment that is recognised internationally as *essential* for clinical work in insomnia rather than PSG. In other words, the complaint of insomnia, systematically summarised on a night-to-night basis, is the most important thing.

You may find it useful if I say a little about the relationship between subjective experience and objective sleep pattern, as measured by PSG. There are different sub-types of insomnia and we will be learning more about these in Chapter 3. One of the more common ones used to be called *psychophysiological insomnia*. In this form of insomnia, the person's experience of sleep can be confirmed by PSG assessment. In other words, someone with psychophysiological insomnia may estimate that it took 45 minutes to get to sleep and PSG will confirm that they had difficulty with sleep initiation. Similarly, if the problem was staying asleep (a sleep maintenance problem) PSG and self-report would agree that there was a difficulty with wakefulness in the night.

However, you may be already familiar with the common finding from research that people usually sleep longer than they think they have. Indeed, you may have thought to yourself 'it feels as if I hardly slept last night, but I probably slept more than I imagine'. The research literature tells us that people with insomnia tend to overestimate how long it has taken them to fall asleep (sleep-onset latency, or SOL), how long they have been awake for during the night (wake time after sleep onset, or WASO), and that they underestimate the total amount of sleep (total sleep time, or TST) that they have had. This has been taken by some to mean that people with insomnia 'exaggerate' their sleep complaint. Little wonder that many people with insomnia feel that their complaints are not taken seriously. However, this *subjective-objective discrepancy* should not surprise us. People who are normally good sleepers are likely to make very similar 'errors' in estimation on those occasional nights when they sleep poorly. This suggests to me that it is not so much the person with insomnia who is in some way at fault; but rather that the task is actually quite a hard one, and one that good sleepers seldom have to perform. During the night, in the absence of stimulation and activity, time can appear to pass rather slowly (don't you know it!).

Another possibility, which has some support from recent research on insomnia, suggests that the PSG, when scored in the conventional way into sleep stages, may fail to identify more subtle EEG characteristics that form part of the underlying pattern in insomnia. For example, a tendency toward frequent *micro-arousals* or the presence of fast EEG waves (as in wakefulness or light sleep) intruding into sleep may correspond better to subjective experiences of insomnia.

Another line of research has shown that people with insomnia respond to auditory tones played while they are asleep, whereas good sleepers do not. When I say 'respond' here, I mean that – at the level of brain activity – auditory *evoked potentials* can be observed in insomnia, which are not evident in normal sleepers. It's not that people with insomnia wake up, but rather there seems to be greater retained awareness during sleep. Remember earlier I said that maybe it is possible to be awake and asleep at the same time? There is also mounting evidence in animal studies of something that has become known as *local sleep*, where some cortical neurons will sleep while others remain awake at time of stress and fatigue. This is really interesting, and clearly much more research in this area is required.

But I never slept a wink!

'Oh yes, you did' you will have heard; 'Oh no, I didn't' you may have answered, or felt like answering! Hopefully, the sections above can help you to understand how differences can arise in the way people perceive sleep. I want to mention, however, a particular form of insomnia where the hallmark feature is this debate, or I might even say dispute, about whether or not sleep actually occurred.

Clinicians and researchers have come to recognise a disorder that used to be called *sleep state misperception*. In this type of insomnia, the individual remains convinced that they obtained no or hardly any sleep, often over extended periods of time. On the one hand this seems unlikely, but on the other hand, there can be no doubt that these beliefs of excessive sleeplessness are sincerely held, by perfectly sensible and reasonable people.

When this disorder has been studied in the laboratory, sleep patterns that are fairly normal are often found. How can this be? Well, perhaps these are extreme cases of the disparity between different methods of assessment; the subjective-objective discrepancy. But we might just as accurately conclude that PSG is simply not up to capturing the nature of this sleep experience. For these reasons, the American Academy of Sleep Medicine re-named this disorder as *paradoxical insomnia*, to reinforce the paradoxical nature of the problem; apparently sleeping well yet complaining of severe insomnia. Paradoxical insomnia should be a priority for further research looking at sleep microstructure. I feel strongly that this 'diagnosis' should not be misused to criticise people who present with such symptoms.

Let us never forget then that the experience of sleep may be different from the sleep records obtained in a sleep laboratory assessment. Both are important, and they are not necessarily in competition with one another for 'right' and 'wrong'. We need to recognise that the complaint of insomnia is what brings people to the attention of health services. Without that complaint no help will be offered or needed. If we distrusted self-reported complaints, people with depression, anxiety or psychosis would not get treated either. I am sure that given time, and good sleep science, better laboratory measures will help us understand the objective underpinnings of the insomnia problem.

What controls our sleep pattern?

You might be thinking that this sounds like a very important section; and you would be right. 'Better control of my sleep – that's definitely what I need, because it is way out of control right now.' So let's dig a little into the science of the sleep control system.

We now understand that two processes work together to regulate our sleep pattern. One is called the *sleep homeostat*, and this controls *drive* for sleep; the other is called the *circadian timer* and this controls *when* we sleep. You can see these mechanisms depicted in Figure 5, and that the arrows show they interact with each other.

Broadly speaking, the longer we are awake, the sleepier we will become. Extended wakefulness, therefore, increases the homeostatic drive for sleep. In physiology, homeostatic processes are there to restore balance, so sleep reduces the drive for sleep, and wakefulness increases the sleep drive. Much in the same way we become parched if we go without fluid, and homeostatic pressure, in this case thirst, increases as time without fluids increases. Drinking satisfies that thirst and so reduces the drive to drink.

The famous sleep researcher, Dr Bill Dement from Stanford University, California, uses the helpful analogy of the 'sleep economy' to explain the homeostatic mechanism.

With each hour that we spend awake we accumulate an increasing *sleep debt*. In healthy good sleepers this debt is then repaid in full by the night's sleep and they awaken refreshed and back 'in balance' the next morning. The analogy raises the possibility that there are individuals who, perhaps through lifestyle choices or for other reasons, find themselves in a state of chronic sleep debt. Indeed, there may be attitudes within some parts of modern society that encourage such lifestyles and pay scant attention to nature's way of replenishing and restoring the individual. Homeostatic pressure for sleep is, naturally, stronger at the start of a sleep episode than it is later on; and this accounts, for example, for why it is that a nap can make us feel much better. Similarly, some people report waking after a couple of hours of sleep and feeling quite awake and refreshed. The restorative value of these early cycles of sleep appears to be proportionally greater. It is also a reason, of course, to avoid napping because there is the potential there to reduce the homeostatic drive for sleep during the night-time period, which is when we really want it to work for us.

So, let's turn now to the circadian part. You may have heard of the *circadian rhythm*. This is a term used to describe the harmony of the sleep-wake schedule. Other functions apart from sleep, such as body temperature, also follow recognised circadian patterns. We are designed to function in a 24-hour world. The word 'circadian' derives from the Latin words *circa diem*, literally meaning around the day. Sometimes we talk about the *body clock*, meaning pretty much the same thing.

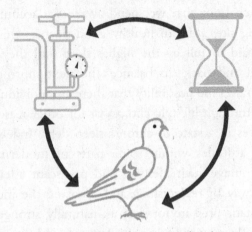

Figure 5: How sleep is regulated

The circadian rhythm takes a little while to become established. During early development an infant's sleep is not organised into day and night phases. Instead an infant will sleep and wake across the 24-hours. By around 6 months, however, the major sleep period becomes concentrated and more settled during the night-time hours of darkness, and there is more wakefulness during daytime/daylight hours. This process of circadian regulation is known as *entrainment*. In this way the body clock gradually approximates to local time. The hormone *melatonin* is largely responsible for the ongoing regulation of the body clock throughout our lives. Melatonin is produced in the brain, in the *pineal gland*. Its production rate is dictated by natural light, so that during hours of darkness (the normal sleep period) melatonin production increases, and as morning approaches and with it the coming of daylight, melatonin production is once again shut down. One of my colleagues in Oxford, Dr Russell Foster, was one of the team involved in making a great scientific discovery some years ago. They found that there are specialised cells in the retina at the back of the eye, called *melanopsin receptor cells*. These cells are sensitive to light and they help to regulate the timing of our sleep. It turns out that our eyes are important not just for our sense of sight, but for our sense of time.

So far then we can see that the sleep homeostat determines our need for sleep, and the circadian system defines the normal timing of our sleep (at night) and the normal timing of our wakefulness (during the day). Of course, there is some natural variation in our daytime wakefulness, and how alert we feel. For example, you will probably be aware of the *afternoon dip* when we tend to feel temporarily rather more tired. Indeed, in some societies it is normal to have a 'siesta' at this time because it also coincides with the hottest part of the day. In terms of our circadian tendencies there is much to be said for that lifestyle!

Circadian regulation, however, is not just to do with our sleep. All major systems in the body have *molecular clocks* that govern the functioning of our organs and their subsidiary functions such as hunger drive. The central *master clock* is situated in the *suprachiasmatic nuclei* (SCN) of the hypothalamus in the brain, and acts like the conductor of the *peripheral clock* orchestra to keep all the organs of the body in tune. I hope this is a useful mental picture and soundtrack. We all know what the cacophony of discordant music might sound like – this is what some people feel like when their sleep-wake system is out of sync with local time, or when their various clock systems are out of sync with each other. The common experience of jetlag is pretty much what I am describing here.

We also know that if we take a single cell – yes one solitary single human cell – and put it in an observation dish with sufficient energy to retain life and function, then that single cell will follow a 24-hour sleep-wake rhythm all on its own. The body clock then is not just a figure of speech; but is an integral part of our very being.

Before moving on from this section, as I was saying before, it is important to note that it is the *interaction* of the sleep homeostat and the circadian timing system that, under normal circumstances, leads to good sleep. Look at Figure 5 again and think of it this way. From the time you wake in the morning, it's as if you begin to build up debt to the sleep banker. Each hour you spend awake is, if you like, sleep deprivation that needs to be repaid. Your sleep debt is growing. However, as the sleep homeostat cranks up, the circadian system interacts with it and holds off repayment. It keeps us awake and alert right across the daytime hours. As evening, night-time and darkness ensue, however, the circadian clock releases its grip on the homeostat. This delivers us into sleep, during which the homeostatic pressure is discharged, the sleep debt is repaid, and we emerge in the morning refreshed for the whole 24-hour cycle to repeat itself once more.

You will see in Figure 5 that I have added another component to the process regulating sleep. Here we have our dove, representing what I call *automaticity*. Apologies for yet another complex term – but it is actually quite straightforward in meaning and it links to what I was saying earlier. People who sleep well usually have absolutely no idea how they do it. Perhaps you have asked them. My point is that the *automatic* nature of this type of 'control' over sleep is crucial to normal, good sleep. The homeostat and the circadian timer, when they are properly adjusted, do their job best without any deliberate control by the sleeper. This is the dove that has landed near one's hand (see page 3). Contrast this with the situation in insomnia where no doubt you are often preoccupied by the sleep problem and its consequences? I call this the *attention-intention-effort* cycle. Your attention is drawn to sleep and to not sleeping, you become deliberate and intentional about your approach to sleep, and you end up trying way too hard, which makes things worse. This is a process that inhibits the natural automatic control of sleep, and it leads to insomnia, when the dove flies away. We will be learning a lot more about this and how to get the right kind of control over sleep using CBT methods.

Why do we need to sleep?

Before I answer this question, let me ask you a different one. What are the bare essentials for life even to exist? Well, I can only come up with four.

These are air, which provides us with oxygen; water which provides us with hydration; food which provides us with nutrients; and sleep, which provides us with function or capability. None of these things is an optional extra in life;

they are all fundamental requirements. In fact, you could survive for three times as long without food, as you could without sleep. We have not, of course, done the experiment on humans, but we do know that experimental animals will die much quicker of sleep deprivation than they would by starvation of food.

Indeed, much of what we know about the importance of sleep comes from the experiences of people who have taken part in selective sleep deprivation experiments. That is, where insufficient sleep, or no sleep, has been taken over successive 24-hour periods. The bottom line is that when people are sleep deprived, they are not able to function properly during the daytime. Figure 6 serves to summarise in a single diagram all that sleep does for us.

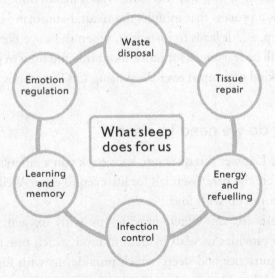

Figure 6: Understanding why we need to sleep

As you can see, even the most basic processes of recovery and body 'maintenance' rely on sleep. We need sleep for waste disposal. I don't mean perhaps what you are thinking of here – although we do of course digest food during our sleep. I'm thinking of toxic waste – and neurotoxic waste in particular. During sleep, there is a deep cleansing of unwanted protein that if not removed could cause both physical and mental problems. Then we need sleep for repair, and for growth. We know for example, that cells are regenerated only during sleep. Research has shown that even equivalent lengthy periods of complete rest don't do that job. So, without sleep, lost or damaged tissue would not be repaired. It really is true that a rest is not as good as a sleep.

Next, in Figure 6, you can see that during sleep our bodies are re-energised for the day ahead. For example, the levels of the energy-carrying molecule ATP (adenosine triphosphate) surge in the early hours of sleep, especially in brain regions that are most active during waking hours. Sleep then acts as a refuelling station; as well as offering a break from the energy depletion of the typical exhausting day. Then you can also see that sleep plays a vital part in what we call immune signalling. We know that lack of sleep reduces the body's production of cytokines which protect us from infection. Antibodies are essential to fight infection and infectious disease, and sleep is nature's way of regulating the body's crucial immune responses. Quite often, we seem to have shaken off illnesses overnight.

Continuing with Figure 6, we also see that sleep plays an enormous role in cognitive and emotional functioning.

Studies have certainly shown that it is not just physical health that is heavily dependent upon sleep.

Let's start here with learning and memory. Lack of sleep impairs our attention and concentration, reduces our ability to multi-task and makes us more likely to make mistakes. Indeed, sleep is closely associated with our ability to be creative and to be sociable. One way of looking at this is to recognise that sleep serves a primary function to make our brain capable of learning, remembering and acting wisely, based on experience. Sleep enables us to perform at our best because our cognitive 'powers' are restored by sleep. Memory consolidation, for example, is dependent on sleep, and research studies have shown that people remember things better after periods of sleep than if they had remained awake.

Sleep also is a primary source of what we call emotion regulation. We can all think how grumpy we are when we need more sleep, but we are also more prone to worry, anxiety and low mood if we are not well slept. I remember my gran telling me that 'things will feel different in the morning . . . what you need is a good night's sleep'. And it's true, there is a recalibration of emotion from impulsivity to reasoned behaviour, and from negativity to positivity following sleep. What sleep offers is a secure platform for us so that during the day we can be free to act on the world as we see it, with all the decisions to make, activities to complete and relationships to manage. During sleep, of course, our minds are given respite from all this 'output' and sleep can do some of its best work to help us re-set and reframe for the next day.

So, as you can see, my simple answer to the question, 'what is sleep for?' is that the purpose of sleep is to make sure we function properly, physically and mentally. I guess that sleep is nature's medicine, so that we can experience a good quality of life. The effects of sustained sleep loss or poor sleep touch almost everything, as you probably know. All the more reason to solve this sleep problem ASAP!

2

Understanding Normal Variations in Sleep

Having thought a bit about normal sleep, I want now to expand on this theme by explaining how sleep patterns can vary, and yet still be 'normal'. There are three main things to say about normal sleep variation. The first is that sleep varies across the night, and in most people across the week. The second is that sleep varies with age and stage in development. The third is that sleep varies from person to person. In this chapter, we will explore these variations and associated topics, like napping, night owls and morning larks, normal triggers to poor sleep, and begin to consider the important question of how much sleep do I need.

Sleeping across the night

We are going to look again at the skyline of the night's sleep. We had an illustration of what the architecture of sleep looks like when we discussed sleep laboratory assessment on page 12 and in Figure 4. This time I want you to go to Figure 7, and to the middle panel showing adult sleep.

This is a simplified hypnogram but once again on the vertical axis on the left we find the stages of sleep, and reading from left to right along the bottom, we find the timeline. You will see here that a notional duration of sleep has been set at 8 hours. This is simply to illustrate what happens over time, rather than to imply that everyone should have 8 hours of sleep!

You can see that in this person, wakefulness quickly gives way to sleep and that there is a rapid progression to deep sleep (N3). This first episode of deep sleep is the longest and deepest of the whole night. The hypnogram has a series of valleys and peaks, with the valleys representing deeper sleep and the peaks lighter sleep. Sometimes these peaks may touch wakefulness. Broadly speaking, deeper sleep dominates the first half of the night and lighter sleep the second half (mainly stage 2). You can also see that at the end of each sleep cycle, there is a period of REM sleep, and that these REM episodes become longer towards morning. This explains why people often feel they have been woken out of a deep sleep if woken up early in the night but may feel that they were simply dozing if woken up towards morning. Similarly, the chances of remembering dreams are greater if you waken during the second part of the night because there is a greater possibility that you were having an episode of REM sleep during that time.

This pattern is pretty much the same on a night-to-night basis, although it is quite normal to sleep a bit later at times (for example on weekends) and also to obtain a greater proportion of deep sleep and dreaming sleep on the night subsequent to a period of sleep deprivation. For example, if

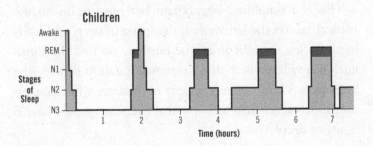

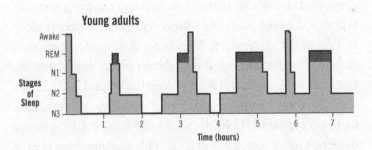

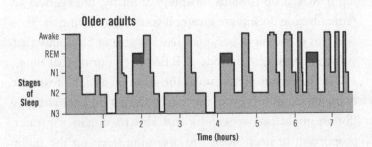

Figure 7: How sleep changes across the life cycle

you are up late for a few nights and have less sleep there will be an increased homeostatic drive towards *recovery sleep*, to repay an element of your sleep debt.

Changes in sleep pattern with age

Everyone knows that our sleep pattern changes across the lifetime. To take an extreme, a newborn baby may sleep 18 hours a day (OK I know – some do not!) whereas older people may feel fortunate if they can put together a spell of 6 hours' sleep. Figure 7 is again helpful here because it illustrates developmental aspects of the sleep pattern and it provides a guide to what might be expected at different ages and stages in life.

The question is – what is similar and what is different in how the phases and stages of sleep express themselves in childhood compared with adulthood and compared with later life? Notice that the broad distribution of sleep remains similar throughout our lives. For example, we always tend to sleep most deeply at the start of our sleep period, periods of REM sleep occur intermittently across the night following periods of NREM sleep, and stage 2 sleep is the most common sleep that we have.

However, maturation and development are also associated with some changes in sleep pattern, and this should really lead us to adjust our expectations of sleep according to the age we are. Few people would deny that children should go to bed progressively later as they grow up, because over time they need less sleep. We regard that as normal, although it is something that everyone has to adjust to! It is equally normal, however, for older adults to sleep less deeply than younger adults, but that may be less widely accepted as a fact of life. There also seems to be a natural *fragmentation* of sleep with age. You will see from Figure 7 that the proportion of NREM sleep that is deep sleep (stage 3) is considerably reduced, and that there is a tendency towards lighter and more broken sleep in later life. By comparison, REM sleep is relatively preserved.

We will see when it comes to the treatment section in Part Two, and you begin to consider your sleep pattern, that it will be important to take into account your own expectations of sleep. In other words, to consider what exactly the sleep problem that you have is, in relation to what might be expected of your sleep just now, and in relation to what might be a reasonable goal for improvement in your sleep.

Taking naps

People often ask me if taking a nap is a good thing or a bad thing. There is no straightforward 'yes' or 'no' answer to that. A number of factors need to be taken into account.

First of all, let me be very clear in saying that people who feel *sleepy* in the daytime, rather than just fatigued, should be prepared to take a nap. If you feel you have a tendency to fall asleep involuntarily, then you are objectively sleepy, and this can lead to risky situations. I am going to describe a 'rescue situation' here; because you have to take responsibility if you are dangerously sleepy. If you are struggling to remain awake while driving or operating machinery, you should stop and take a nap for 10–15 minutes (not necessarily longer). This type of nap, in these circumstances, accompanied by a cup of strong caffeinated coffee is likely to help you temporarily overcome sleepiness. Take the coffee first then take the nap. The nap restores you a bit, taking the edge off your sleepiness, and because the caffeine kicks in after you wake up, the stimulant effect can help you stay awake.

But I hear you say that you thought that you should not take naps during the day, and that you should reserve your sleep for night-time? This also is true. In the paragraph above, I was referring only to the special circumstances where there is danger associated with falling asleep. In insomnia, sleepiness of this type is not usual, and if it is a problem for you, and is not simply because you are working too hard and giving yourself little time to catch up on sleep, then go to your doctor and get your sleepiness checked out. Returning to insomnia, people more commonly feel tired or fatigued and in need of rest, rather than sleepy during the day. There is an important difference here. Feeling tired or like you lack energy is not the same thing as struggling to remain awake. As a general rule, therefore, if you are not actually sleepy then my recommendation is that you do try to avoid taking naps outside the night-time sleep period. Your goal is to become a good sleeper and we know that sleeping during the daytime can reduce the body's drive for sleep at night. If having a nap is so much part of your routine that you do not want to give it up, then you should restrict the nap to a single period of no more than 15 minutes, and take your nap absolutely no later than the early evening. Let me repeat, however, that if you can avoid taking naps, you should do so.

There is no denying that some people can take naps and still be good sleepers at night, but if you are suffering from insomnia, naps in all likelihood just add to the problem.

As with sleep itself, there are also normal variations in napping, from person to person, and across different cultures. Napping is also more common in older adults than in younger adults, in part due to lowered activity levels, and in part to a weakening of the circadian rhythm which controls sleep and wakefulness. Although I am fairly confident that napping does not in itself cause insomnia, I am certain that it does not solve it either. There is more information on napping and how it relates to CBT for insomnia in Part Three.

Good and poor sleepers

Some people are familiar with the notion of 'good sleep' or 'poor sleep'. You hear individuals describe themselves as 'poor sleepers' and you hear others describing themselves as 'good sleepers'. But it is also very common for people never to have thought about this distinction. Or at least this can be so for the good sleepers. This is consistent with the idea of automaticity that I mentioned earlier – we don't really think about sleep . . . until it's not there when we need it!

It is better to think of sleep in *relative* terms, not in absolutes or categories, like good and bad. I think this difficulty in differentiating is even clearer when we consider the idea of the 'good night' or the 'bad night'. The truth is that most people have a mixture of these. Admittedly, the good sleeper generally sleeps well, and the quality of that sleep over time is not usually broken. However, occasional 'bad nights' do occur. Similarly, the person with insomnia reports sleeping poorly much of the time. I tend to operate on the basis that people with insomnia have at least three 'bad nights' every week, but even they also have some nights when their sleep is adequate and refreshes them as it should.

We can see then that sleep may be variable, for all sleepers, although this variability is much more pronounced in insomnia. But why would people who are good sleepers sometimes have bad nights? I think there are three reasons. First, people who sleep well do not keep to perfect routines. We live our lives in the real world and that inevitably involves some variability in how we spend our time. Changes of life-style pattern, even temporary ones, have some consequences for sleep. Secondly, the same experiences that contribute to the broken or inadequate sleep of the person with insomnia do also affect, from time to time, people who normally sleep well. Take for instance stress. Everyone knows what it is like to lie awake at night with your mind racing. But I think there is also a third reason. It may be that the occasional night of poor-quality sleep, or of diminished sleep, has a useful function for the good sleeper. Such occasions may provide the sleep homeostat with the opportunity to 'flex its muscles', and to demonstrate that it is working properly by bringing sleep back into line on subsequent nights. It's as if recovery after a bad night's sleep happens naturally for the good sleeper so they tend not to overthink it, and just assume it will happen.

I can sense that some of you reading this are probably quietly seething away about my suggestion that people with insomnia have occasional good nights of sleep! Some of you may feel that you have not had a decent night's sleep for years! I respect your sentiments, because I have heard this so often. My response here would be that I am talking in relative terms. All I am saying is that you are likely to have some nights that are better than others. It is unusual for a person with insomnia to have an identical sleep experience every night. Thinking about your sleep in black and white terms is not likely to help you. You need to begin to see the shades of grey.

Others of you may agree that you have a mixture of sleep experiences – and this can be one of the most frustrating things about insomnia. Perhaps you have thought 'why is it that sometimes I can sleep reasonably well, but I just cannot get myself into a proper pattern?' Never knowing which night is going to give you a reasonable sleep leaves people very frustrated . . . and wakeful! The unpredictability of insomnia can be part of its menace, every bit as much as the relentless aspect of being stuck with a chronic problem.

I want to make one other point here. Just as there are people with larger feet or smaller feet, or with larger or smaller appetites, or faster or slower metabolisms, there are people who seem to be better sleepers than others. Similarly, just as there are people who were short for their age in childhood but became tall adults, so there are people who were poor sleepers when they were younger and better sleepers when they were older. Maybe not everyone is going to be the best sleeper! It is worth considering that it may be part of normal variation that some people will be more fortunate than others in the strength of their sleep pattern. That is not to say that your sleep cannot be improved – but just bear in mind that it is a fact of life that not everyone is the same.

What is sleep deprivation?

I have mentioned the term *sleep deprivation* several times already. It certainly sounds punitive! Indeed, throughout history, systematically depriving people of sleep has been used as a form of punishment or torture. We have discovered that the body and the mind can survive much better without food than it can without sleep, so one can only imagine that deliberately depriving people of sleep would have dramatic effects.

The scientific investigation of the effects of sleep deprivation, however, is relatively recent, although much of this work was done several decades ago. It is interesting that, even when sleep deprivation experiments were conducted under controlled laboratory conditions, ethical concerns arose about these experiments because of the risks attached to them. Nowadays this type of research is seldom undertaken, except in very limited circumstances. Nevertheless, it was through carefully controlled sleep deprivation research that we began to better understand the functions of sleep. The specific functions of the different stages of sleep became a bit clearer through studies on selective sleep deprivation. For example, not allowing people to have REM sleep led to disorganisation of mental processes such as perception, thinking, learning and memory.

But are people with insomnia sleep deprived? As we have learned, sleep is regulated by the brain, and even when this regulation is in some way upset, brain mechanisms work hard trying to prevent us from getting into a perilous state of sleep deprivation. We have learned that as we go longer without sleep, so the drive for sleep increases, and we are forced to sleep. Insomnia is not really a disorder of sleep deprivation. It is more helpful to think that people with insomnia carry a burden of unsatisfactory sleep. Insomnia is often associated with a persistent feeling of sleep insufficiency and with daytime impairments to mood and quality of life.

I could sleep anywhere!

You might be wondering why I have put this topic in a section on normal variations in sleep. The reason is that I find there is quite a lot of individual variation in the ability to sleep in different circumstances. Some people can 'sleep on a pinhead', in any situation. There are people who seem to be able to sleep right through a long-haul flight, who adjust more quickly to new time zones, who can sleep comfortably in a camp bed . . . and so on. And of course, there are others who find that they can only sleep under particular circumstances, often only in their own bed, and only if they get to bed by a certain time, and so on. These people sometimes talk about 'catching the moment', or say that they become anxious if they get to the stage that they are 'beyond their sleep'. Most of this I would put down to individual variation – people are different – no more, no less, and in that sense, it does not really require too much explanation.

What is interesting in insomnia, however, is that sometimes people are actually able to sleep better in unfamiliar environments. As mentioned earlier, this might be because they associate their own bed so strongly with lying awake that they have a kind of conditioned response to it and are unable to fall asleep. Another explanation might be that in an unfamiliar environment they really do not expect to be able to sleep and, because they are not so concerned about trying, they become more relaxed and are able to drop off.

Of course, there are people with insomnia who have problems sleeping in any situation. For some it is simply worse on vacation, or when staying with friends. It is not uncommon in my experience for people to dread, and to avoid, what should be enjoyable times because they worry that their insomnia is going to interfere with their plans. This is yet another example of how intrusive insomnia can be.

Owls and larks

I am sure we all know what an owl is: someone who has a tendency to be up at night. This is the kind of individual who comes to life late in the evening and into the small hours, often having energy and alertness at times when most of us are beginning to feel really quite sleepy. By way of contrast, the lark is someone who is at their best in the morning, preferring to be up early and to make the most of the early part of the day. The owl is not usually good in the morning and the lark is not usually good at night.

People who have one or other of these tendencies simply have a stable sleep-wake phase position that is slightly different from the average. Sometimes this is referred to as *circadian preference*. However, it's not so much that they are choosing their lifestyle; rather, there is now research evidence to show that there are genetic predispositions to having the trait characteristic of 'eveningness' (the owl) or the trait of 'morningness' (the lark). Usually people adapt to their body clock tendency, and often they quite like it; they make it work for rather than against themselves. Sometimes, I see this expressed in their occupation. For example, I have seen a number of people who have been radio presenters, doing late night shows, and it suited them really well because they were the kind of people who thrived on being up late. It was a different matter for them when they were put on to morning shows!

Another reason to mention these so-called *clock types* or *chronotypes*, is that they can interact with insomnia. Take 'owls' as the first example. They don't feel sleepy until later than usual, so it is quite possible that the combination of a biological tendency to remain alert until late (let's say 1 a.m.) with the desire to get to sleep (say) at 11 p.m. will express itself in 2 hours struggling to get to sleep and worrying that you cannot get a full night's sleep to prepare you for an 8:30 a.m. work start. Owls might also struggle to waken up and feel sleepy into the mid-morning at work, but this is not because of insomnia – it is because they are still in their biological sleep period. Morning people, the 'larks', have exactly the opposite problem. They can fall asleep very easily because their biological sleep window is early – let's say 9 p.m. However, they can struggle to sleep through until morning. They naturally waken early, but they can complain of not having had enough sleep, perhaps because they stayed up late in order to be sociable.

Table 1: Average sleep requirements at different ages

Age range	Typical sleep requirement
Newborn	A newborn baby may sleep up to 18 hours. At first sleep is taken across the 24 hours with no dominant sleep period. By 4–6 months sleep becomes more consolidated at night.
Young child	Toddlers sleep up to 12 hours at night and normally also sleep for 1½–2 hours during daytime naps.
Child	By the age of 4 years daytime naps will normally have stopped and the child will sleep 10–12 hours at night. This sleep requirement reduces to around 10 hours during the early school years.
Teenager	During adolescence sleep duration is normally around 9 hours. There is some variation in when sleep is taken, e.g. it is common for young people to stay up late and sleep on into the morning.
Young adult	The young adult typically requires 8-9 hours' sleep.
Adult	Sleep requirement in terms of total sleep time does not vary greatly during the major part of adulthood. Around 7–8 hours is average.
Older adult	In later life sleep is less consolidated at night, with 6-7 hours being typical. However, there is a tendency once again to 'top-up' with some daytime naps.

Social jetlag

I'm not sure if you will have heard of social jetlag? Nothing to do with air travel! It's a term that has been used to describe the differences in sleep timing that can emerge between workdays and 'free' days. For example, a person may have to get up at a fixed time on weekdays for school or college or for a day job, but may have a much later (lagged) wake and rise time on weekends when they are free to follow an underlying sleep tendency towards later rising, or to catch up on sleep lost during the week. Social jetlag can of course interact with your chronotype, so it's worth taking this into consideration as you attempt to understand your personal sleep pattern in relation to your lifestyle.

How much sleep do I need?

I am sure we are all familiar with the perils of interpreting average figures! If you are a parent you will be familiar with having measured your child's height and weight against what are called normative values, or norms for short, in order to check that everything is progressing as expected. Although norms give the impression that there is a right answer, more careful consideration helps us to recognise that in fact we are usually talking about a normal range. To take a different example, that of intelligence, the average IQ may be 100, but this certainly does not mean that most people have an IQ of 100 . . . or that they should have! What it does mean is that the normal range of IQ is around 100, so that scores between 90 and 110, or even 80 and 120, would be considered to be normal.

Table 1 provides some information on what is regarded as the normal range of total sleep time at different ages. You can inspect this table and compare for your own age group and see what you think. Of course, even when a value falls outside the normal range, this does not actually mean that there is necessarily something wrong. For example, you might expect that most adult males will be between 5' 6" and 6' 2" tall, but this does not mean that being 5' 3" or being 6'4" represents a problem. Here we have to introduce what is known as the *normal distribution*. That is, outside the middle part of the normal range there is *always* a smaller number of individuals with lower and higher scores. Exactly the same applies to sleep. There are people who are constitutionally *long sleepers* and people who are constitutionally *short sleepers*. Inevitably, these individuals are at the outer margins of the normal distribution, but it does not necessarily mean that their sleep pattern is pathological. For example, if a person is a short sleeper but has no adverse consequences, we would have to suppose that a relatively small amount of sleep is in fact sufficient for that person's needs.

I'm sure though you are coming back to the question . . . but how much sleep do *I* need? How do I find that out if I can't just read it off a chart? This is a great question, and it is actually one of the things that you will discover through following the CBT programme!

Triggers to poor sleep

I wanted to end this chapter on normal variations in sleep with a brief mention of 'triggers' to poor sleep, because this topic forms a natural bridge to considering insomnia. Everyone has some nights of sleep disturbance, and often there is an identifiable triggering event or situation. For example, people commonly report disruption to their sleep pattern when there is something important on their mind (e.g. a test or a test result, or an argument), when they are sleeping in an unfamiliar environment (e.g. near a busy road, in a tent), or when they experience some kind of upsetting life event (e.g. unemployment, medical concern). Indeed, it seems that any changes in life circumstances have the capacity to disrupt sleep, even when these are positive life events that we might be looking forward to (e.g. a holiday, a social event).

What I am describing here is a normal process. Sometimes it has been called transient insomnia or acute insomnia and here it is normal for the insomnia to be short-lived. That is, poor sleep is a temporary experience for most people. In the usual course of events we might expect that good sleep will be reinstated once the stressor or the life change has passed, or when we adjust to the stressor. One of the research challenges that we face in the study of insomnia is why it is that some people recover so well and resume good sleep patterns whilst others develop persistent insomnia even though it may at the start have been triggered in a relatively normal way.

So, let us go on now to explore insomnia in greater depth.

3

Understanding Poor Sleep and Insomnia

So, what is insomnia?

Now that we have had a chance to think about what sleep is, and why it is important, let's turn our attention to understanding insomnia. This is an important step towards finding ways to overcome it.

The word *insomnia* has its origins in Latin, where *somnus* was the word for sleep, and *insomnus* was the word for sleepless. *Insomnia* became the English language version of being sleepless, and probably describes how you often feel! Like many other words in everyday use, people talk about themselves as *having insomnia,* but *insomnia disorder* is also a medical term that has a specific meaning. Are they the same thing? The same would apply to someone saying that they feel depressed; because depression is also a medical disorder.

There are three main *diagnostic classification systems* that we use internationally to diagnose insomnia as a disorder. These are the *Diagnostic and Statistical Manual of Mental Disorders*, the 5th edition of which (DSM-5) was published in 2013; the *International Classification of Sleep Disorders*, the third revision of which (ICSD-3) was published in 2014, and the *International Classification of Diseases*, the 11th edition of which (ICD-11) was published in 2022. These large reference books are what clinicians use to decide if a person has a *sleep disorder*. For our purposes, we are most interested in the diagnosis of *Insomnia Disorder*. Several *criteria* have to be met for a clinical diagnosis.

The characteristics of insomnia

At this point in the book, I am simply summarising the main features of insomnia that are consistent with the diagnostic criteria. When we get to Chapter 6, I will walk you through an assessment of your own insomnia problem.

As you can see in Table 2, insomnia is a difficulty getting to sleep or a difficulty staying asleep . . . or both! To meet the criteria for insomnia disorder, this sleep complaint also needs to be present three or more nights per week. In other words, the insomnia has to be a regular feature of the individual's experience and in this sense has to be typical of their sleep pattern. The next criterion concerns the severity of the sleep disturbance. Here you will see that it needs to take more than 30 minutes to fall asleep (on a minimum of three nights per week of course) for the individual to have insomnia of the sleep-onset latency (SOL) type. For the sleep maintenance (WASO: wake-time after sleep-onset) type of insomnia the difficulty needs to include more than 30 minutes of wakefulness during the night. In my clinical practice, people commonly have both SOL and WASO difficulties, that is they have at least 1 hour of wakefulness during the night, either at the beginning or during their sleep period. Indeed, many have 2 or 3 hours of wakefulness during the night, most nights.

Another way that we sometimes look at the severity of insomnia is to consider the individual's sleep efficiency (SE), a term I mentioned earlier. A cut off point of SE = 85 per cent is commonly used in clinical practice and also in research to define significant sleep disturbance. In other words, on average 15 per cent or more of the time in bed is spent wakeful. To give an example, if you normally sleep for a grand total of 6 hours per night but are in bed for around 8 hours, your sleep efficiency is 75 per cent, and you are spending 25 per cent (2 hours) lying awake in bed each night.

Table 2: The diagnosis of insomnia disorder

The complaint	Difficulty getting to sleep or staying asleep
Its frequency	Three or more nights per week
Its severity	Sleep-onset latency (SOL) or wake time after sleep-onset (WASO) more than 30 minutes
Its duration	Present for at least 3 months
Its effects	Marked distress; impairment socially and/or occupationally; other important consequences

The duration criterion I have given you in Table 2 is that insomnia must have been a problem for 3 months or longer.

This indicates *persistent insomnia*, which is sometimes called *chronic insomnia*. The majority of people with severe insomnia complaints have had the complaint much longer than that. In my clinical practice it is commonly around 10 years, as an average, so people usually have no difficulty meeting the duration criterion!

The final criterion in Table 2 refers to the effects of the insomnia upon the individual. This is important, because it is often the consequences of insomnia for the person that leads them to seek treatment. It may be that the effects are primarily social. This could be in terms of irritability or low mood, or other aspects of interpersonal functioning; or it could be that the effects are more upon productivity in everyday life, in which case concentration and alertness may be problematic. Either way there is usually considerable distress associated with the knock-on effects of insomnia. For the person with insomnia, an unsatisfactory night is often followed by an unsatisfactory day. Sound familiar?

As I said, we will look at your particular insomnia profile later on. We will figure out whether your sleep problem meets night-time and daytime criteria for insomnia disorder using a clinically validated tool called the *sleep condition indicator*.

Insomnia sub-types

I have already mentioned the *sleep-onset* and the *sleep-maintenance* types of insomnia. I have also explained that there can be a *mixed* sleep-onset and sleep-maintenance problem. I want to add here that some people are the *early morning awakening* (EMA) type. This is a specific example of sleep-maintenance, where the person doesn't get back to sleep at all after the final wakening. So, they wake at say 4 a.m. and then remain awake until they get up. Whatever the sub-type may be, we now just simply use the term *insomnia disorder* to describe the condition.

But what about the circumstances where insomnia may have some connection with a health problem? Well, in years past we might have asked the question about whether the health problem was the primary difficulty. Certainly, at times of physical illness, sleep can become disturbed. Also, pain or discomfort associated with a medical disorder might cause problems for restful sleep at night. Other examples might be drawn from the psychological and psychiatric field, because insomnia can be associated with mental ill-health. Anxiety disorders and depression come immediately to mind. If you are stressed, anxious or depressed it is quite likely that you will sleep poorly.

Nowadays however, we take the view that both problems should be treated. That is, for example, the insomnia and the depression; or the arthritis and the insomnia. This is because we know from research studies that insomnia and a poor sleep lifestyle makes people vulnerable to developing physical or mental illness in the first place. It doesn't make sense any longer to see sleep problems as just a consequence of something else. Besides, if you have a physical health problem or a psychological problem, it does not mean that your insomnia cannot be improved using CBT. There are countless studies that show that sleep can be helped by CBT in people who have these co-morbid physical or mental conditions.

Finally, there are some people whose insomnia is connected to the use of sleep medications. Normally this is in individuals who have been long-term users of what we call 'hypnotic' drugs. In these circumstances, the habitual taking of sleeping pills in itself has become a problem. The individual with *hypnotic dependency* finds it extremely difficult to stop taking sleeping pills, and when such attempts are made the insomnia problem magnifies considerably, leading to them going back on the sleeping pills. If you feel this could be you, you should seek professional assistance and perhaps follow a structured programme to taper off and withdraw the medication gradually. The CBT programme described in this book may be helpful to you, but you do need to recognise that sleeping pills themselves can cause some insomnia effects. For example, some medications for sleep cause *rebound insomnia* when you cut them down or stop using them. This temporary worsening of the sleep pattern can be distressing, and in some cases can last for several weeks. I have provided a separate chapter in Part Four to give you more information about sleeping pills, and also about other medications that can interfere with your sleep.

In summary, then, insomnia is a persistent disorder involving regular sleep disruption and its associated daytime effects. It may occur on its own, or it may be associated with other disorders or other problems. My CBT programme should help you with your insomnia, whatever type it is, but you should certainly seek other advice too if you have any concerns about your physical or mental health or your medication.

Other types of sleep problems

I have now introduced the sleep diagnostic systems to you, with a focus on insomnia, but there is a wider range of sleep disorders within the DSM-5, ICSD-3, and ICD-11 classifications. Some of these disorders have similar symptoms to insomnia, so it is important that you check out that your problem is not some other type of sleep disorder. To help you with this I have included in Chapter 6 what I call a 'screening procedure' to help you see if you may have any other types of problems. These can sometimes be there alongside insomnia, just like a medical or mental health problem could be. I have also written a separate chapter (Chapter 16) in Part Four, on recognising and managing other common sleep disorders.

How common is insomnia?

There have been a lot of studies that address this question and they provide us with a good indication of how common sleep problems are in the community at large.

Of course, you will be familiar with the argument that statistics can be used to tell us anything! It will be of little surprise to you, therefore, when I say that there is quite a wide range of estimates where insomnia is concerned. Much depends on the question that was asked in the particular

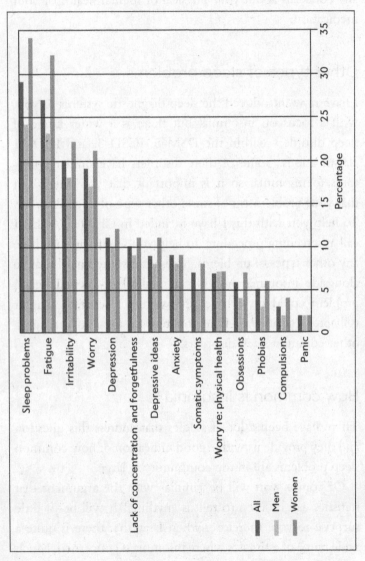

Figure 8: Insomnia is a common problem

survey. For example, if people were asked 'do you some-times have difficulties sleeping?', most people would answer 'yes'! Likewise, if people were asked 'do you think you are a poor sleeper', up to half of the general population may say that they are; and the other half may say that they are not. Apart from the question that is posed, another factor which influences the results of such studies is how many people are approached, and whether or not they are representative of the general population. Needless to say, a poorly conducted study is not going to give us very good information.

The most reliable of these kinds of studies of insomnia are ones that have included questions related to the diagnostic criteria I outlined for you in Table 2. Many such studies have been conducted and from these we can estimate that around 1 in 10 (10 per cent) of the adult population has persistent problems getting to sleep and/or staying asleep. This figure rises to 1 in 5 (20 per cent) of adults over the age of 65 years. You will see, therefore, that insomnia is a very common problem indeed!

To illustrate this further I thought it would be helpful to compare insomnia with some other common problems. In Figure 8 I have presented some information from a large study conducted 20 years ago in the UK, so this shows that insomnia has been a recognised problem for a long time now. This was a study investigating a whole range of mental health symptoms in the general population. Here the researchers were interested to find out how common symptoms of depression, anxiety and so on were in order to help plan appropriate services in primary care (community-based general practice). You should note that because the questions focused on symptoms rather than having a disorder, the percentages shown are much higher than the numbers of people with clinical problems. Nevertheless, what we can see is that sleep disturbance and fatigue were by far the most commonly reported symptoms amongst UK adults. This was true for adults of all ages, whether male or female, and regardless of the region that people lived in the UK, or their ethnic background. The graph demonstrates quite clearly the relative importance of sleep disturbance compared with other mental health complaints that people commonly need help with.

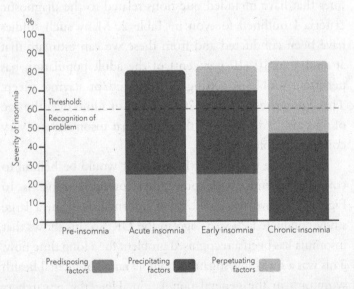

Figure 9: Predisposing, precipitating and perpetuating factors

So, you will see that you are not alone in having insomnia! Far from it. Insomnia is an enormous public health problem, affecting the quality of life of countless millions of people around the world.

From occasional to persistent insomnia

It remains a bit of a mystery why insomnia might develop from being a short-term problem, or an occasional difficulty rearing its head from time to time, to a persistent or chronic problem. But we have some important clues!

The late Dr Art Spielman from the City College of New York proposed a model of insomnia development and persistence that can be useful here. As we can see in Figure 9, we may assume that everyone has some degree of vulnerability or *predisposition* to develop insomnia, just as one might presume that we have a level of predisposition to develop any other kind of problem. For one individual that predisposition may be higher, say because of a family history of the problem or having a less well-regulated circadian rhythm, or because of a tendency towards anxiety. As the model suggests, however, that predisposition on its own would not normally lead someone to develop an insomnia disorder. Dr Spielman proposed rather that insomnia presents, first of all, at an acute level when *precipitating* or triggering factors are sufficient to reach a certain point. We can think of a wide range of such factors that might be relevant here, including temporary changes in our sleep environment, or our home environment, or work-related stresses, illness, acute anxiety and so on.

However, under normal circumstances we would expect that when those temporary, triggering factors diminish again, a good sleep pattern would be reinstated, and the symptoms of insomnia would decline. The model goes on to suggest, therefore, that *perpetuating* factors are required if an insomnia disorder is going to persist. We can imagine that becoming concerned and anxious about sleep itself could be a powerful perpetuating factor for insomnia. Similarly, in response to such concern, the person with a developing insomnia might disrupt their own sleep patterns further by making behavioural changes to sleep routines. For example, it is tempting to try to catch up on sleep by going to bed early or sleeping in late, but this might just lead to a drop in sleep efficiency rather than a gain if it means that an even longer time is spent lying awake in bed.

There is also a line of research suggesting that the *thoughts and beliefs* that people with insomnia develop about their sleep, and about their sleeplessness, can contribute to persistent insomnia becoming established. A common example would be that people with insomnia develop the concern that how they feel during the day is largely a result of how they slept the night before. Therefore, they try to anticipate and to control their sleep at night. This thinking pattern becomes associated with anxious thoughts about sleep that are *arousing* and also counter-productive to sleep itself, and also counter-productive to daytime relaxation.

A model of insomnia development

Some of my own research has investigated the process of *automaticity* that I described earlier. Have a look back at

Figure 5. You will recall that good sleepers are normally quite unaware of how or why their sleep pattern is so well regulated. It just seems to happen . . . as it were automatically. They don't really think much about it. I want to go into a more detailed explanation of automaticity so that you can understand how the *inhibition* of this process could lead to insomnia developing and to the dove of sleep flying away.

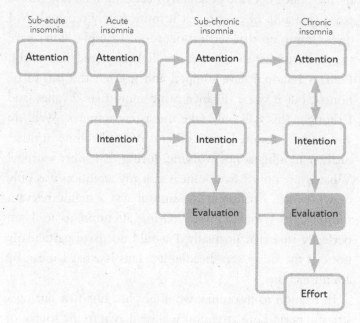

Figure 10: Model of insomnia development

Let me start by explaining why it might be that some people go on to develop a persistent insomnia (after a short, acute episode of sleeplessness) whereas others seem to resume normal sleep patterns. There is a concept in psychology known as *attentional bias*, meaning that our attention is drawn towards objects and events in our environment that are particularly relevant to us. Let me give you a simple example.

One wintry November evening when I was driving home, I realised that one of my car headlamp bulbs had failed. Now, during the previous winter, I had been stopped by the police because of a faulty headlamp bulb and had to pay a fine and, of course, get it immediately repaired. As I drove home on that second occasion, I simply didn't have the opportunity to get the headlight repaired that night. Perhaps I should have stopped and just left the car, to be honest, but it was a distance of no more than 2 miles, and I thought this will only take me a few minutes. Well, do you know, I counted seven other cars that had one or other of their headlights not working during that short journey! What is my point? My point is that my attention was only drawn to this because at the time it was a highly relevant stimulus, so I found myself paying attention to it. I am perfectly sure that normally, I would not have particularly noticed the other cars' headlights. This is what I mean by attentional bias.

In relation to insomnia, we might imagine that during a stressful period our attention will be drawn to the source of that stress (e.g. unemployment) and to its immediate consequences (e.g. financial problems). The acute insomnia that might go along with such a stressful episode may not need any special explanation. At this stage, although we may be aware of not sleeping well, we may not pay much attention to sleep, because our attention is taken up elsewhere . . . and even if we do think about sleep, we may not think it requires a separate solution. However, there may be a transfer of attention to sleep at some point, perhaps if the insomnia gets worse, or if the original stressor reduces but sleep does not improve spontaneously. Focusing on insomnia can then lead to further problems with sleeping.

We have now conducted many attentional bias experiments and have found that people with insomnia do indeed respond more attentively, even to very subtle 'cues' associated with sleep and sleeplessness. Another reason we believe that this model may be important is that studies on attentional bias in other areas of psychology suggest that these vigilant 'response biases' develop in situations where we feel under some kind of *threat*. For example, people with dog phobias scan their environment and seem to notice more dogs than people who do not have this phobia. The number of dogs out there doesn't change but their sensitivity to their presence changes hugely.

But why would insomnia pose a threat? It's not like a fear or a phobia − is it? Well, I think that the inability to sleep actually may be fundamentally threatening because of the biological importance of sleep. To be unable to sleep, or to believe that you are unable to sleep, perhaps sparks off a primitive feeling of threat . . . of danger. Remember that there are only four things that are fundamental to survival. If you felt you were starved of oxygen, water or food, that situation probably would trigger your basic threat instincts and make you hypervigilant for a solution. It might be the first thing in your mind. Might it not be the same for sleeplessness? On top of that, if you had always slept well in the past you may feel very, very puzzled and threatened by the idea that something you previously took for granted, and never had to do anything about, or even to think about, has now become a problem!

So, let's consider the model in a bit more detail by looking closely at Figure 10. You start off on the left-hand side. You are not sleeping as well as you used to and your attention at this point is drawn to the thing that is upsetting your sleep; the stress factor or whatever it is that's on your mind. I have called this *sub-acute insomnia* because it has just happened and is not severe at first. However, in the next column, headed *acute insomnia*, the initial thing that disrupted your sleep has begun to recede, but you have noticed that you are not sleeping well, so you have become more attentive to your sleep. I suggest here that you develop perhaps for the first time an *intentional process*. You did not previously pay much attention to sleep, nor did you have particular sleep intentions . . . but *now* it feels like you need to have a solution. The intentional process is a *planning* process where you begin to think through options and decide on what to do about your developing sleep problem. The intention to sleep is another step along the way to converting what used to be an unconscious, automatic process into a deliberate plan. It is as if you have swapped your car's automatic gearbox for a manual version. You have taken over more of the controls. Consequently, automaticity is inhibited even more . . . and, of course, attention is further heightened because you become even more aware of sleep and sleep-lessness in your life. You are on the edge . . . the beginning of the end of automatic sleep. A sign that the dove is getting restless!

So now both attention and intention are switched on. You are rapidly losing your sleep's automatic pilot. One possibility is that your plan works out well and that your sleep recovers quickly. In this case automaticity would be re-established (back on autopilot) and attention and intention would be switched off again. The dove would settle, and you would as usual neglect even to notice that it was sitting there. However, there is also the possibility that you take the first steps towards insomnia proper; here I call it *sub-chronic insomnia*. This happens if you become really concerned that your sleep is not getting better, that your insomnia is still there.

It is likely that this *evaluative process* will directly inhibit the automaticity of sleep, for two reasons. First, scrutinising your sleep performance in this way will focus more (not less) attention and intention. Second, evaluation introduces both a cognitive and an emotional component to the develop-ment of insomnia. The cognitive part engages the reasoning part of the brain – 'what's going on, how is this happening; I need to make sense of this; I need to solve the problem'. The emotional part kicks in when we think about success/failure . . . 'my sleep isn't getting better; I don't know how to sleep; things are going downhill; if I can't sleep, I won't be able to cope at work; I feel I'm losing control'. This last point is important because the model of how good sleep is regulated, that I proposed in Figure 5, is that good sleep 'control' is automatic . . . yet here we have the incorrect and unhelpful idea developing that sleep *should be* under deliberate control and that you need to fix it.

You can see the culmination of all this in the furthest right column in Figure 10. An *effortful process* becomes engaged in what has now become a *chronic insomnia* disorder. We already have attention, intention and evaluation switched on. What happens now is that we increasingly try to sleep – we put in a big effort . . . we do everything we can . . . leave no stone unturned . . . we use all the resources we can find . . . *to try to get sleep*. This effortful process is driven by emotion, maybe even desperation. Of course, feedback from the evaluative process is likely to be negative – it isn't working – so attention, intention and even more effort are likely to become heightened further still. Needless to say, all this focus and sleep effort puts the final nail in the coffin of automaticity. The dove has flown. Everything is now anything but automatic. Our work on the development of the *sleep effort scale* suggests that sleep effort is highly relevant to the experience of insomnia. You will learn more about this scale and how to use it later on.

I believe that it is in the *context* of sleep intention and sleep effort that the person with insomnia ends up doing things that make it very unlikely that good sleep will be able to return spontaneously. With sleep automaticity damaged, the sleep homeostat and the circadian timer become more vulnerable to our emotions and to our behaviour. For example, in my experience people with insomnia often make their problems worse, not better, by changing their sleep patterns back and forth. Most commonly, they end up spending too much time in bed in relation to the amount of sleep they are getting, so sleep efficiency plummets, and the experience of *conditioned arousal* in bed increases. What I mean by this is that the bed and the bedroom become associated with wakefulness; to the point where even going into bed triggers anxiety and delays sleep. I am sure you have experienced the frustration of trying your best to sleep. However, malfunctions in how the homeostat and the circadian timer operate are, ironically, perhaps the consequences of you trying too hard to put things right. All this hopefully is beginning to make sense of why a cognitive and behavioural (CBT) approach is likely to be effective for chronic insomnia.

In summary then, I think that this model of *preoccupation with sleep* may represent a *critical* difference between the good sleeper and the person with insomnia. I hope that you can see that there is a lot of interesting work going on to understand why and how insomnia develops. Later on, we will think not just about this model, but about other factors that interfere with sleep. I'm sure you will find a good explanation that makes sense to you, and that the CBT which flows from that will offer you an effective solution to get your sleep back to its natural best.

The doctor's dilemma

It is not uncommon for people with insomnia to feel misunderstood! To a good sleeper there is nothing particularly complicated about getting to sleep, so they may not understand, and do not know what to suggest. That's not to say that people do not sympathise. Everyone has experienced occasional bad nights of sleep . . . enough to know that it is a horrible experience.

More often than not, however, the physician does not really know what to suggest either. Very often people with insomnia are left with the feeling that they just have to live with it themselves. Sometimes it is suggested that they might be depressed, and on occasions this is correct too. Sometimes the insomnia will be defined by saying what it is *not*. For example, 'I don't think you've got sleep apnoea', as if to say that what you *have* got is *only* something else – something else called 'insomnia' . . . which you probably already knew.

I do not mean to be cynical here. I am just reporting what I hear time and again. But let me provide a corrective to the tone of my comments. I believe that physicians have an extraordinarily difficult task when it comes to trying to give advice about insomnia disorder. Their dilemma is this: they are presented with a distressed person who has a persistent and intrusive complaint, for which they usually have no effective treatment immediately available.

Traditionally, doctors have prescribed medication for insomnia. However, sleeping pills are recommended *only* for short-term insomnia, not persistent insomnia, and prescription of medication is particularly discouraged in older adults whose bodies are slower to break down the chemical compounds in the drugs. All of the so-called 'hypnotic' drugs are relatively unproven over the longer-term, so we do not really know what benefits they have to sleep with protracted use. Certainly, many people who are in the habit of taking sleeping pills find that they continue to have significant difficulties getting to sleep or staying asleep. The beneficial effects of the medication also tend to wear off, requiring either a higher dose or a different hypnotic. In some cases, this can lead to a dependency problem, especially if there are *rebound insomnia* symptoms associated with the medication. Your doctor should be aware of the benefits that can be associated with occasional or very short-term use of various sleeping pills, as well as their limitations and the way they may interact with other medications.

Over many years now, there has been increasing interest in the use of melatonin as a sleep aid. In some countries, this can be bought over the counter in a pharmacy, and in other places, it is prescription only. As I mentioned earlier, melatonin is a naturally occurring hormone in the body that seems to be closely coupled with the timing of sleep. Unfortunately, when taken in tablet form, melatonin does not seem to be a solution for insomnia. It has more of a role to play with circadian rhythm sleep-wake disorders. I will mention these in Part Four.

There is really only one other prescription option. That is to prescribe drugs that are not licensed for insomnia but may still have a useful effect. This is called *off label prescribing*; and is used most often when the side-effect of the drug (which is licensed for some other condition) causes sleepiness. An anti-depressant drug might be given for example, either because there is a suspicion of an underlying depression associated with the insomnia, or because the anti-depressant drug happens to have a sedative side-effect when taken at night. The all-too-common practice of prescribing an anti-depressant in the absence of depression, however, remains controversial. The most commonly used drugs for this purpose are in a group called the 'tricyclic anti-depressants'. However, there are few controlled clinical trials of these drugs for the purpose of treating insomnia and this is a matter of ongoing debate and concern amongst sleep medicine specialists internationally. Likewise, pills for epilepsy, for allergies, for pain or for hypertension are sometimes prescribed for insomnia if they have sedating properties. All of this is because the doctor is trying to help, though there's little scientific evidence that they will be effective.

The treatment with the best evidence of success for chronic insomnia is, of course, CBT. Indeed, clinical guidelines worldwide recommend CBT as the first-choice treatment that should be given to patients with persistent insomnia. The doctor's problem here is that CBT is often not readily available or accessible to their medical practice. *Clinical Psychologists*, or others trained in CBT methods as applied to insomnia, are normally needed to treat people with insomnia effectively, and these specialists can be a scarce resource.

Fortunately, there is growing interest in the field that has become known as *Behavioural Sleep Medicine*. The American Academy of Sleep Medicine, the European Sleep Research Society and other sleep societies worldwide now have specialist sections for those interested in and certificated in behavioural sleep medicine practice. There is a dedicated Society of Behavioural Sleep Medicine too. There are also more training opportunities than there used to be. At the University of Oxford, for example, in 2016 we started an international Master's Programme in Sleep Medicine, that is fully online, so clinicians from around the world can enhance their training and skills. I very much hope that assessment and treatment services for people with insomnia will expand both in association with established Sleep Centres and Sleep Laboratories, and in the community at large. The advent of the digital age also offers an exciting new treatment option in the form of digital CBT for insomnia.

In the meantime, hopefully you will find that the CBT methods I have laid out in this book will work for you.

4

Understanding the Consequences of Insomnia

Simply having a bad night?

As we now know, insomnia is a disorder of getting to sleep, a disorder of staying asleep or a disorder that involves both of these problems. It is important to start this chapter on the consequences of insomnia, therefore, by considering the impact that insomnia has on the *experience* of sleep itself.

It is extremely unpleasant to lie awake at night, unable to sleep, and hoping either that sleep will come soon . . . or perhaps that morning will come soon! People with insomnia have this negative experience very regularly, and it becomes very demoralising. Don't you agree?! Just in the same way as having bad experiences at work, or in a close personal relationship, can lead you to feel low, or helpless, or frustrated, so you can get similar feelings with repeated experiences of inability to sleep.

If this were a work situation, you might want to change job or to retrain. If a personal relationship, you might want to avoid the person involved. When we are stuck in a bad situation, we usually want to improve it, to change it, or to get out of it. Similarly, people with insomnia *so much* want things to be different. Have you been caught up in that vicious cycle of sometimes reluctant acceptance, other times fervent efforts to overcome sleeplessness, and then again . . . hopelessness, when the insomnia just will not go away? Sometimes people say to me that they become so anxious as bedtime approaches that they cannot bear the thought of yet another night of restless wakefulness.

For all these reasons, you might think it a bit odd that the clinical diagnostic criteria for insomnia require that there are also daytime consequences to a poor night-time sleep. As if to say, 'so what, you don't sleep at night . . . but you get by – right?' Personally, I think it *is* a big deal to sleep so badly, without patients feeling they have to justify their insomnia by demonstrating how tired or miserable they feel 24 hours a day. These days we talk a lot about 'quality of life' – but do we really just mean quality of waking life? Surely, we should recognise that life is made up of daytime and night-time and that satisfaction and fulfilment in both of these areas is important.

Not infrequently, in the exchange of pleasantries when meeting someone I have never met before, I get a further glimpse of how the world at large views the importance of a good night's sleep. Once people find out that I research insomnia problems and their treatment they often say things like 'I absolutely hate my sleep being disturbed, it's the worst thing' or 'I couldn't cope if I didn't get my sleep'.

Even for good sleepers, having the occasional bad night is pretty much universally a memorable experience! The other response I get, of course, is 'Oh that's really interesting because I have had this problem sleeping for years . . . !'

Suffice to say that sleep is such a fundamental thing and not being able to sleep is no trivial matter . . . for any of us!

Sleepiness and fatigue

Of course, it doesn't end there for people with insomnia, and the clinical diagnostic criteria are correct in that regard. Night-time wakefulness is bad enough in itself, but it normally comes with other baggage. The first item that most people mention is sleepiness or fatigue. When you haven't slept well at night you are quite likely to feel not so fresh, not so rested during the day.

I have used both these words, sleepiness and fatigue, not because I think they are synonyms, but in fact because I think it is important to understand the difference between them.

Fatigue can be a numbing, disorienting, even depressive kind of feeling – the 'can't be bothereds' if you like. Fatigue is both a physical and a mental experience. Muscle and mind alike seem to resist our best efforts to engage them when we are fatigued. But you can feel fatigued, or perhaps you prefer the terms 'tired' or 'weary' (I think they are about the same thing), without actually being likely to fall asleep.

The tendency to fall asleep, particularly to fall asleep involuntarily, is at the extreme end of the spectrum. Fatigue does not mean that we are literally unable to stay awake – that is a different thing. That is sleepiness. People with insomnia seldom are so extremely tired during the day that they cannot help but fall asleep. Excessive sleepiness of this kind is more likely to be the result of sleep deprivation or of a sleep disorder such as narcolepsy or obstructive sleep apnoea. Consequently, if patients I see at my clinic tell me that they simply cannot stay awake, that they fall asleep at the drop of a hat even when they don't want to, then I would most likely commence further clinical investigations.

Pervasive and enduring weariness – the feeling that 'my get up and go has got up and left' – now *that* is typical of insomnia!

Problems concentrating

This feeling that everyday tasks are an effort often reveals itself as a problem with concentration. In psychology, we talk in terms of 'information processing'. What we mean is that in order to interact with the world, we need to be able to *perceive* (see, hear, sense) what is going on, and we have to be able to *attend* to what is going on. When we are alert and our mind is sharp, recognising and paying attention to relevant information comes quite naturally. However, when we are tired, information processing becomes more strained, and involves the brain in more work. This is usually what people mean by concentration – that is, the struggle to keep focused on something coupled with the sense that the particular task should not normally take that amount of effort.

People with insomnia often comment that they feel they 'miss things', that they are not quite 'on the ball'. It is as if the brain's information processing system is not working as efficiently as it should be. Because a fundamental purpose of sleep is to maintain good quality daytime alertness, it should not surprise us to find that insomnia has this kind of impact. Sometimes people complain that they are more forgetful because of their insomnia. This may be down to the concentration problems – things were not taken in properly in the first instance. Alternatively, it may be harder to remember, that is to retrieve information from the memory store. It is as if their whole mental apparatus has slowed down. This sluggishness in thinking and reasoning is one of the ways that insomnia has consequences for the day.

Becoming irritable and moody?

The other main area of complaint associated with the daytime consequences of insomnia, is how poor sleep can affect our mood. Have a look again at Figure 8. There we have it – sleep problems, fatigue and irritability – the three most common mental health symptoms.

When we become irritable it is often because we are tired, or our attention span is short, or we are finding it a struggle to do something that we think should normally be a simple task. We might find that we are reacting more impulsively to situations and are not in that regard quite our usual selves. So, you will see the connection between our mood and our ability to think clearly. In my clinical work, people often tell me that they are easily provoked, or on a 'short fuse' if they have had insufficient sleep. This is made even worse if they have a busy schedule during the day and feel that they are failing to perform to their usual standards.

A sense of nervous edginess can also accompany insomnia. This may be part of the body's defence mechanisms against tiredness, by making the person rather hyper-aroused during the daytime, in order to stay alert. We see this clearly in young children, as they become more tired and bedtime approaches. We say they are 'fighting sleep'. A very similar phenomenon often occurs in insomnia.

On becoming depressed

This is an interesting and important one. Does insomnia cause depression? . . . or is insomnia simply a symptom of depression? I honestly think that the answer is both of these things.

There is a great deal of scientific evidence now that insomnia is associated with depression, and that it often comes *before* depression. Indeed, if we combine all the data from research studies, we find that having persistent insomnia for a year or more can double your risk of developing depression for the first time, or for becoming depressed again if you have had it before.

When you think about it, would you expect that poor air quality, impure water or a poor diet would have no health consequences? Sleep protects us from emotional disorder by regulating our mood; so, it follows that poor sleep over an extended period of time may have consequences too, and one of the first casualties can be that we become depressed. Some people may be prone to develop an anxiety disorder, and others may find that alcohol dependence becomes greater.

I hope I am not alarming you here, but it is important for you to understand what clinical research tells us about the relationship between sleep and mood. You might be thinking it is bad enough to have insomnia, I don't want to become depressed as well. Alternatively, it may be that this helps to explain how you have been feeling. The good news is that insomnia is treatable, and if it is a risk factor for the development of depression, it is a treatable risk factor.

It is also clear from research that insomnia is a very common symptom of depression. That is, people who become depressed for whatever reason, usually don't sleep well. Clinical guidelines now recommend that whatever comes first, insomnia or depression, both should be treated. This is because they both merit treatment, and can be helped; but also, because insomnia does not always recover as quickly as other depressive symptoms and can continue even when the depression lifts. A good way to think about this is that there is a two-way interaction between mood and sleep – and this extends to other mental health problems too; anxiety and alcohol use, but also other problems such as post-traumatic stress and psychosis.

If you are feeling depressed, it is important to figure out what role insomnia might be playing, and to get advice on how best to manage the depressive and insomnia elements. I should mention too that sometimes the sleep issues in depression can be more at the *hypersomnia* end of things:

sleeping much more than usual. Either way, restoring your sleep to a healthy schedule is likely to be helpful.

Coping and everyday life

Thinking about the consequences of insomnia in terms of symptoms (tiredness, mental slowing, irritability, depression, etc), however, does not tell us the full story. The main impact of insomnia upon the daytime is on how it affects *what we are able to do*. People are concerned about their concentration because they feel they are likely to make mistakes at their work. They are concerned about their irritability, because it is affecting family life, and so on. It is this interference with daytime functioning, in personal, social and occupational situations, that often leads people to seek professional help. Living with the experience of poor sleep at night, may have felt barely tolerable, but add to this these intrusive effects upon daytime quality of life, and you have a problem that is hard to ignore.

Consideration of how we cope during the day, however, raises a very interesting and important issue. It is not easy to draw a direct line between sleep and daytime performance. For example, we can and do become irritated for other reasons apart from lack of sleep. It may be hard to concentrate if we are taking on too much, or if we are distracted by things round about us, or if we are in too much of a rush. You will find out that analysis of what we call 'attributions', the connections between cause and effect that we tend to make, is one of the therapeutic ingredients of CBT.

Insomnia and its effects on the family

In many respects insomnia is a lonely experience. You may have felt, in the middle of the night, as if you are the only person in the world who is awake! It can also feel lonely in the sense that your bed partner may be a good sleeper; or it may be that you experience loneliness associated with living alone and not having someone to share a bed with.

I find that other people in the family are commonly affected in some way by a patient's insomnia. A common concern of people who have sleepless nights is that they may disturb their partner's sleep, or the sleep of others in the household. So, on top of the anxiety about not sleeping itself, they have this added worry to deal with. They may lie in bed unsure if they should get up. If they are out of bed, they may be unsure if they will manage to get to sleep if they go back to bed. In this way, there is often a big discrepancy between the sleep pattern of the person with insomnia and others at home – going to bed at different times, falling asleep at different times, waking and rising at different times. This can cause disruption and tension. Indeed, it is very seldom that I see people whose partner also has insomnia. You might think it fortunate if insomnia were to be synchronised in this way, because people might then be able to support each other. Then again, that may be the reason why I do not see them at my clinic!

It is clear that insomnia can be disruptive for other people in the family. It can also cause problems in other ways. There may be limited understanding about insomnia, or sympathy towards it, at home. At times, insomnia certainly can be a source of relationship strain. Couples may be sleeping in separate beds or separate rooms. Partners who sleep well may find it hard to believe that you have not slept. Because they have been asleep, it may be natural for them to assume that you have been sleeping too! There is also the fact that the family may have to deal with the consequences of your insomnia in terms of your fatigue and mood.

Effects of insomnia on social life and working life

As a general rule, people who have persistent insomnia simply do not feel at their best to take part in things. Consequently, the other areas that are particularly affected are work and social participation.

The work situation can be affected both by concentration difficulties and emotional factors. Things are harder to do after a bad night's sleep. It can be tiring to have to fight off fatigue constantly, and the more we are aware of feeling tired, the more tired we often become. Insomnia can also affect the workplace. Some recent studies suggest that people with insomnia have more time off work either through being late in, or through sick leave, than people who sleep well. There is also the problem of 'presenteeism'. That is, you may be there at work – literally be present – but not be able to engage as productively as you would do if you were well slept. In clinical practice, I sometimes see people pulling back from promotion possibilities, especially those that involve additional responsibility, because they fear that they cannot give their work the attention it deserves. Insomnia causes a loss of potential and a loss of fulfilment that would otherwise be open to these people.

Emotional factors play a part not only in the office or factory, but also in our informal contacts with people in social and leisure settings. Generally, people expect us to behave consistently, and that can be hard if our mood is up and down or if we are on edge through lack of sleep. Sometimes, patients tell me that they have cancelled even their most enjoyable commitments and pastimes due to lack of energy, and fear of upsetting their friends by appearing distant or temperamental. Indeed, one of the things we know from research studies is that lack of sleep causes us to act more on impulse, perhaps making rash judgements, and this can become problematic in relationships with others. Everyone is different of course, but many people with insomnia have social lives that are in some way restricted.

Insomnia and physical health

I have already described how insomnia can be a risk factor for mental health problems, notably depression, and for day-to-day coping, for relationships and for work performance. But we now know that physical health problems are also more common in people with persistent insomnia.

Over the past 10 years, many research studies have been conducted to investigate the relationship between insomnia, as a specific type of sleep disorder, and medical disorders or risk for the development of a disorder. From these studies, it seems that insomnia may contribute to the development of type 2 diabetes, cardiovascular disease and to health vulnerabilities such as obesity, reduced immune functioning and hypertension. It may be that insomnia lowers the individual's threshold for ill health, meaning that they may be somewhat more illness prone. The research suggests that people with insomnia who are also short sleepers (6 hours or less) are at particular risk of developing poor health; and some studies have even reported lower life expectancy in people with persistent insomnia.

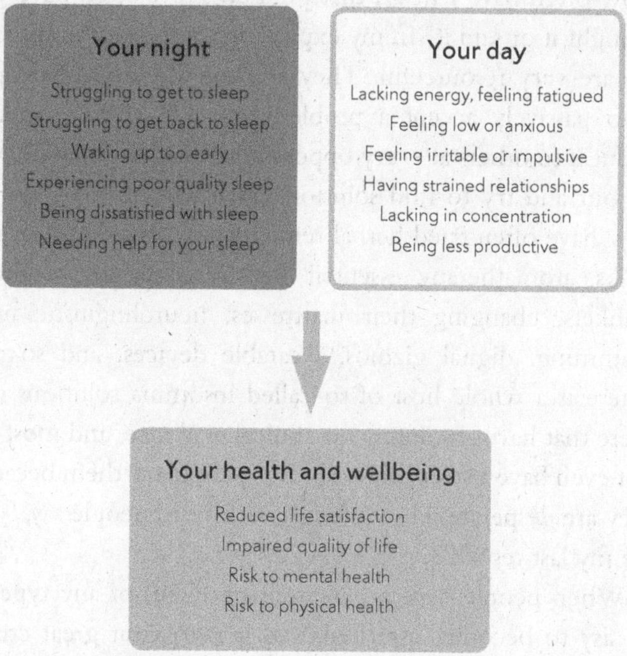

Your night

Struggling to get to sleep
Struggling to get back to sleep
Waking up too early
Experiencing poor quality sleep
Being dissatisfied with sleep
Needing help for your sleep

Your day

Lacking energy, feeling fatigued
Feeling low or anxious
Feeling irritable or impulsive
Having strained relationships
Lacking in concentration
Being less productive

Your health and wellbeing

Reduced life satisfaction
Impaired quality of life
Risk to mental health
Risk to physical health

Figure 11: How insomnia affects our lives and our wellbeing

All this goes to show that insomnia is not a trivial problem.

In Figure 11, I have summarised information in diagrammatic form, to illustrate how insomnia may impact on your life. As can be seen, consistent with what we have been exploring, insomnia affects both your nights and your days, and it potentially affects your mental health as well as your physical health.

Insomnia is well worth trying to overcome!

But I have tried everything already!

How often have I heard that phrase?! How often have *you* thought it or said it? In my experience, people with insomnia are very resourceful. They are not the kind of people who passively accept a problem; nor do they complain about it to others at every opportunity. Rather, they usually go out and try to find solutions. Apart from medications, they have often tried herbal remedies, various diets, special milks, aromatherapy, essential oils, homeopathy, weighted blankets, changing their mattresses, neurolinguistic programming, digital gizmos, wearable devices, and so on. There is a whole host of so-called insomnia solutions out there that have absolutely no clinical evidence, and most do not even have a scientific basis. But people try them because they are desperate. How often have I heard people say, 'you are my last resort!'?

When people have a persistent problem, of any type, it is easy to become dispirited, and it is to your great credit if you are the kind of person who has kept on trying to find a solution. The very fact that you have this book in your hands right now is testimony to the fact that you or someone close to you has thought that it might be helpful. Now that you have come to CBT, I hope that this will provide the answer you are looking for. It is just about time to move on now to practical matters like assessing your sleep and setting about improving it. But why should CBT offer you an answer when everything else has failed?

Let me explain why this book is about CBT, and why CBT offers you something new and effective. There are three possible sources of evidence we can look to, to evaluate the benefits associated with any form of treatment.

The first source is anecdote. The personal testimony of people who have found something to be helpful can be influential. The premise underlying the power of anecdote is 'it worked for me, it might work for you'. This is of course a logical possibility . . . but there are usually no data to tell us whether it worked for anyone else, or to compare outcomes with those for whom it did not work. Anecdote, therefore, is not a reliable source of information because it does not deal with probability, but only with possibility. I am not quibbling with the 'no harm in trying' school of thought. I'm simply stating that anecdotal evidence is an extremely limited form of evidence.

The second source of evidence comes from marketing. There are many products in the sleep solutions marketplace that claim to alleviate or cure insomnia. Some are branded as health products or lifestyle products and so they appear to have credibility. We all want to be healthy and improve our lifestyle, and the fact that they are permitted for sale to the general public suggests that they are safe and effective. Let me also mention sleep apps here. The vast majority of these rely on endorsement by users, on social media, and on company claims about helping you sleep. Again, as with the anecdote, I am not saying that products that rely on what is sometimes called the 'wisdom of the crowd' and on market claims do not help some people. What I am saying is that they do not offer any scientific evidence concerning probability of benefit for someone who has a persistent insomnia problem that requires a treatment solution.

The third level of evidence is what we rely on in scientific study to establish the effectiveness of any treatment for any health condition. This is where products and procedures are systematically tested in *randomised controlled trials* (RCTs). It is normal to test firstly against chance variation over time – that is the possibility that some people will improve anyway at random; and secondly, to test against the placebo effect – that is the possibility that some people will improve simply because they hope or believe a treatment will work. The amount of true benefit associated with a treatment, therefore, is established only when the effects of time and placebo have been carefully extracted. It is on the basis of studies such as this that not only I, but all leading world authorities on sleep, and all independent clinical guideline development groups, recommend CBT as the best treatment for persistent insomnia.

CBT, and component parts of CBT, have been extensively evaluated using RCT methods over the past 35 years.

Hundreds of such trials have been conducted worldwide and have been published in the scientific literature. Data from these trials have been pooled to determine the overall probability of benefit associated with CBT. The good news is that CBT is regarded, on the basis of this large body of evidence, as the *treatment of choice for persistent insomnia, by all leading clinical, medical and scientific authorities worldwide.* Unlike sleeping pills, the benefits are not only short term. Two-thirds to three-quarters of people with even the most persistent insomnia have been found to obtain lasting clinical benefit from CBT. My goal is to help you become one of them.

PART TWO

ASSESSING YOUR SLEEP AND YOUR INSOMNIA

PART TWO

ASSESSING YOUR
SLEEP AND YOUR
INSOMNIA

Introduction to
Part Two

In Part One we considered some general questions such as what is sleep, why does it matter, what is insomnia and how does insomnia affect us? Here in Part Two, I want to help you think about your own sleep, and about your own sleep problems. So, I am going to take you through a detailed assessment of your sleep. However, before we even begin to see where the problems might lie, I feel it's important that we get some basics in place that will serve as a platform for everything we do together. I call these the five principles of good sleep health.

5

The Five Principles of Good Sleep Health

What do you expect to read when you come across a heading like this? Most likely a set of 'sleep tips', some 'do's' and some 'don'ts'. However, the five principles are *not* about the usual suspects – things like caffeine, comfortable mattresses, ideal bedroom temperatures, the use of devices and the like. Such things, typically known as *sleep hygiene*, are rather superficial. After all, sleep is fundamental to every living organism. Cats and dogs, birds and butterflies don't sleep well because they leave their smartphones in the living room, or because they cut down on their Americano intake! So, don't you think it unlikely that those things in themselves will be crucial to how humans sleep well? What, as you will see, is crucial is that like all animals, we protect our sleep. This is where our failures in sleep hygiene demonstrate the core failure which is about the place we give sleep in our lives.

I'm thinking of principles that are fundamental to developing a healthy and *trusting sleep mindset*. Let's get the principles of the trusting sleep mindset right, let's base the principles upon the best knowledge and the best science, and then the practices of a healthy sleep lifestyle can follow on. I want to help you to get the most out of your sleep. We all absolutely need to get the benefit of this precious part of nature's provision.

Likewise, although the five principles relate to your mindset, they are not in themselves CBT, far less a stand-alone treatment for insomnia. Indeed, the five principles apply to everyone, whether or not you have a sleep problem. That's one reason I'm placing them up front here, even before we assess your sleep. These principles contain truths for everyone, all of the time. So, I do hope that the five principles will be provocative, even inspiring perhaps, and will encourage you to take a deeper interest in overcoming your insomnia as we go through this book together.

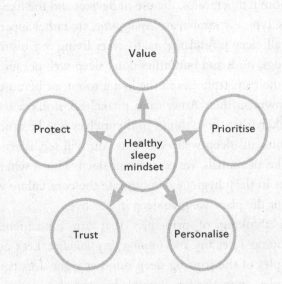

Figure 12: Five principles

First principle: Value your sleep

When we strip things right down to the most basic of life's essentials, when we explore the very foundations of our needs as humans, what do we find? We find just four central physiological ingredients that give us the capability to live our lives. We need oxygen so we can breathe, we need water so we are hydrated, we need food so we are nourished, and we need sleep so we can function. Sleep plays the central role in the renewal and repair of body tissue, in metabolism and the clearance of waste, growth and development, infection control, learning and memory, and in the regulation of our emotions.

Perhaps you didn't realise that sleep is quite so crucial? The quality of our daytime alertness, energy, productivity and mood is greatly dependent upon sleep. Think of how you would be the next day if you hadn't slept? If clean drinking water and sufficient food are important, so is having enough good quality sleep. Don't cut corners where sleep is concerned. It can be damaging to health in the long-term, and that shouldn't come as any surprise. The same would be true if we were malnourished. But sleeping is also a bit more like breathing. It's not something you can choose to do. You can't hold your breath – well not for very long! Likewise, you can't switch sleep on; you have to set the scene with the right attitudes and behaviours and then it will happen naturally. Sleep is so important that it will happen automatically. It's a biological thing. This is why it is also impossible to stay awake. Indeed, one of the dangers of not getting enough sleep on a regular basis is that you will fall asleep without intending to. The first principle of establishing healthy sleep then is that you need to take sleep seriously. You need to *value* it as highly as a fresh water supply, good food and the air that you breathe.

Second principle: Prioritise your sleep

This follows from a mindset that takes sleep seriously. You should *prioritise* getting your sleep. In other words, not just warm thoughts and good intentions, but action. Prioritising means that you will more often put sleep first, or at least higher up the list, when it comes to making choices of what you want to do. At times, this will mean letting go of things that you might actually prefer to do. This can be difficult. Who likes to be the first to admit they are tired, or to stifle a yawn? Or to be the first person to leave the party, especially if it just seems to be getting going! It's possible that you will feel a bit guilty or that you are letting other people down. Social pressures, actual or virtual/online, come into play. Yet it can be done. We can choose to prioritise our sleep.

In other quarters we have become used to managing these pressures. For example, expressing our personal dietary preferences is much easier than it was before. In the best scenarios, there will be respect rather than mockery in demonstrating self-discipline about being true to our values. We want to value our sleep – right? Remember that the purpose of sleep is to deliver health, wellbeing and ability to function during the day. A well slept, well rested you is going to be better for everyone. It can be difficult to prioritise your sleep of course when you don't have control of the situation. You could be working shifts, and your night-time might inevitably have to be given over to work. You might have a new baby at home; and so, I hear you saying, 'I wish!' to the idea of prioritising your sleep. I do hear you. On the other hand, if it's hard for you to choose how and when to sleep, I suspect that you will even more wholeheartedly agree with the need to prioritise sleep when you get the opportunities to do so. So, the second principle is about making commitments and setting behavioural goals to create the necessary space for sleep in your life.

Third principle: Personalise your sleep

If you are following along with this then hopefully you are now considering how you can value your sleep and are thinking of actions that you can take to prioritise getting your sleep . . . but how much? . . . and how much is enough? This is probably the most common question that I get asked! And then people ask about quality of sleep – is quality of sleep not every bit as important as quantity of sleep? So . . . my third principle is about figuring out and understanding your *personal sleep requirement*, and then satisfying those personal needs. I say personal, because we are not all the same. It never ceases to amaze me that we seem to think everyone should follow exactly the same sleep pattern. Our other physical characteristics, appetites and preferences differ.

How much sleep do you, personally, need? How do you figure it out? That's actually a question with a simpler answer than you might have thought – you figure it out by trial and error. That is actually how we learn most things in life. For example, if I were to ask you the question 'how do you know your shoe size?', would you not think it a bizarre question? Did someone tell you what it ought to be? Have we all got the same shoe size perhaps? You find the shoe size you need by trying on different sizes until you find the one that fits most comfortably. Personalising your sleep is the same; it's simply about experimenting to find the best fit. How long do you need to be in bed to get enough sleep? If you are willing to experiment to discover your best 'sleep window', I fully expect you will figure it out.

Part of this personalising is also about your 'chronotype'. That is, when is the best time for you to go to bed and to get up? People who are natural night owls will tend to feel sleepy later in the evening and to feel sleepy later into the morning. Morning larks are the opposite, feeling sleepy earlier in the evening and waking up alert early, first thing in the morning . . . or even before first thing! Accept who you are. Personalise your sleep by getting the sleep that you require, and when you require it. If you do this, you will begin to find that the amount of sleep you need, and your experience of sleep quality, will begin to match up.

Fourth principle: Trust your sleep

If you have experimented a bit and given sleep the

right-sized space or sleep window at the right time for you, the main thing to do next is to *trust* your sleep to get itself into a good pattern. It helps if you can use the same pattern and timing for sleep during the weekend as on weekdays. Remember that sleep is a natural process that the whole animal kingdom can rely upon. So, once you get your pattern and timing right, you want to let your sleep needs and your sleep pattern drive you, rather than you trying to drive them.

Let me let you into a secret – good sleepers are actually not 'good at sleeping'. They are usually not doing anything at all except trusting and expecting sleep to come. In fact, to be honest, they seldom even think about it. Honestly, nobody is hiding anything from you about how to get to sleep, or to get back to sleep if you wake up! Trusting your sleep involves resisting the temptation to grab at solutions, trying this and trying that as if you are walking some kind of tightrope. This just heightens anxiety, leads to preoccupation with sleep, and will make you feel precarious and desperate. I so often hear people talking so passionately about sleep. More than anyone perhaps, I totally get that. But I have to tell you, as you probably already know, it doesn't work to become frenetic and to overthink the whole thing.

If you can't sleep then just get up for a while, accept that, and go back to bed when you feel sleepy again. Please remember too, that you can still experiment until you get the shape and timing of your sleep right. Trial and error, as I said before, but informed by what you have already tried. Be prepared to try going to bed for shorter periods of time too so that you are properly sleepy when you settle down; and get up at the same time each morning. All this strengthens the sleep-wake rhythm and helps to establish a pattern you can trust. Keep a note of your experiments if you like. I would rely on data, on evidence from what works and what doesn't.

Fifth principle: Protect your sleep

Finally, let's think about how you can *protect* your sleep, by avoiding or preventing things that can cause some upset to sleep. These things may seldom be the cause of poor sleep, but nonetheless you should think them through and address what might be relevant to you. Protecting your sleep falls into three categories. First, there are lifestyle factors. The stimulant properties of caffeine and nicotine tend to delay the start of sleep so caffeinated drinks are best avoided in the evening; and bear in mind that most e-cigarettes still contain nicotine! Alcohol also disrupts sleep, particularly during the second half of the night; and heavy meals too close to bedtime can lead to restless sleep. Exercise is a good thing, but it's best to have a wind down time before you retire so I suggest exercising early to mid-evening rather than immediately before going to bed. Winding down your activities and responsibilities is a good idea! Probably the biggest thing in the lifestyle category in fact.

Second, there are environmental factors. Again, experimenting is a way to discover the bedroom environment that suits you. Sleep generally likes cooler and darker, but you can try things out – not too hot or too cold, not too bright or too dark. Also, not too noisy or too quiet. Try to keep the bedroom well ventilated though and make sure your bed is comfortable. Third, I want to say a few words about devices and gadgets. These are a mixed blessing, I think. It's good to take an interest in your sleep, but not good to overanalyse it! Also, most devices that claim to measure sleep don't publish scientific evidence, particularly on people who sleep poorly. So, I would be wary of the accuracy of the information you get from watches, wearable wristbands, and sensors in the bedroom. Finally, the problem that I see with tablets and smartphones is not so much that they are sources of light in the bedroom, but that they are triggers to remaining awake and alert so you can read information, engage in social behaviour, or play games that act as a recruiting sergeant for vigilance rather than sleep! It makes sense to keep your bedroom as a sleep place if you really want to protect your sleep.

Summary

I would urge you to value, prioritise, personalise, trust and protect your sleep. Following these five principles of sleep health will enable you to be your best you. None of us can do without sleep; and why on earth would we ever want to? Certainly, there are pressures on our lives that can make sleep hard to come by, but we need to figure this out. It's important that we do, because sleep is nature's great healer and provider, not just for us but for all living things. I know that you are having sleep troubles that need more attention than this, so we are moving on next to assessing your sleep, but I hope my five principles have helped to set us up for success!

6

Assessing Your Insomnia Problem

What kind of condition is your sleep in?

To start our assessment, I want to take a quick temperature reading as it were, to see what kind of shape your sleep is in at the moment. Have a look at Figure 13. This is the sleep condition indicator or SCI for short. It is a measure I developed a number of years ago around the time the DSM-5 diagnostic criteria for insomnia disorder were published. I wanted the SCI to be able to test for insomnia, but at the same time to be as user-friendly as possible. Fill it in now. As you can see there is also a version available online. Hopefully it is fairly self-explanatory.

I expect you will have a number of items checked in the grey area to the right of the SCI because this indicates where the sleep problems lie. You will also see that items at this end are scored lower. This is because on the SCI a high total score indicates better sleep and a low total score indicates poor sleep. What is your score out of 32? You can also recalculate your SCI on a 0-10 scale. What shape is your sleep in?

Item	Score				
	4	3	2	1	0
Thinking about a typical night in the last month . . . 1. . . . how long does it take you to fall asleep?	0–15 mins	16–30 mins	31–45 mins	46–60 mins	≥ 61 mins
2. . . . if you then wake up during the night how long are you awake for in total? (add all the wakenings up)	0–15 mins	16–30 mins	31–45 mins	46–60 mins	≥ 61 mins
3. . . . how many nights a week do you have a problem with your sleep?	0–1	2	3	4	5–7
4. . . . how would you rate your sleep quality?	Very good	Good	Average	Poor	Very poor
Thinking about the past month, to what extent has poor sleep . . . 5. . . . affected your mood, energy or relationships?	Not at all	A little	Some-what	Much	Very much
6. . . . affected your concentration, productivity or ability to stay awake?	Not at all	A little	Some-what	Much	Very much
7. . . . troubled you in general?	Not at all	A little	Some-what	Much	Very much

Finally . . .	I don't have a problem / < 1 mo	1–3 mo	3–6 mo	6–12 mo	> 1 yr
8. . . . how long have you had a problem with your sleep?					

Scoring instructions:

Add the item scores to obtain the SCI total (minimum 0, maximum 32)

A higher score means better sleep

Scores can be converted to 0–10 format (minimum 0, maximum 10) by dividing total by 3.2

Item scores in grey area represent threshold criteria for DSM-5 insomnia disorder

A free online version, with built-in score convertor, is available at www.sleepio.com/sleep-condition-indicator/

Figure 13: The sleep condition indicator

We have gathered data on very large samples of people now and I can tell you that the average score on the SCI is 15. Are you scoring 16 or more (better sleep than average) or below 15 (poorer sleep)? I wouldn't be surprised if you are poorer, maybe by quite a bit. After all that's why you are reading the book!

In Figure 14, there is a detailed diagram with data summarised from 200,000 people who have completed the SCI. What you see are called box plots. It may look a little complicated, but notice that the average sleep condition in men is a bit higher than in women, at all ages. Also notice that typical sleep condition reduces as you get older. Like other things, sleep ages a bit!

If you like, you can find and mark yourself by sex and age-group on Figure 14 and see where your SCI score lands. The boxes represent a range above and below the average for each group. Maybe you are below average but still in the box, or maybe you are further below average than that. Don't be concerned if you are. It's not unusual for us to find SCI scores down to low single figures in our studies on insomnia. And the good news is that CBT can really help even if your sleep is in very poor shape!

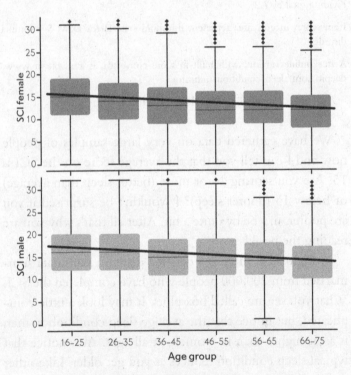

Figure 14: Sleep condition indicator scores in women and men across different age groups

Your insomnia profile

You will have noticed in filling out the SCI, that I am interested not just in getting a total score but also in understanding your insomnia profile. There were questions about your sleep pattern, about your sleep quality, about the effects that poor sleep is having on you, and about the severity and duration of your problem. If you look back at how you scored the items on Figure 13, you will see that profile, with some ratings more to the right (worse) than others. Some items might be less problematic, and it's good to pay attention to those too.

I want you now to complete the detailed profile in Figure 15. You can look back to what you put down for the SCI because some of the items are similar. Figure 15 has an example profile (for Charlotte) already completed in the left panel. This is to show you what to do. In the example you can see that Charlotte has a mild (once or twice per week) but persistent (lasting more than 3 months) sleep-maintenance insomnia (problems with wakenings, but not with getting to sleep at first) and associated daytime effects of fatigue and mood disturbance.

I suggest that you now complete your profile by circling the arrows and the descriptions in the furthest right column that best describe your sleep problem. You might want to write your profile down in the box on page 122.

Night-time (My problem is that...)	Check (→)	
I can't get to sleep at the start of the night	→	Sleep-onset Insomnia
I can't stay asleep during the night	→	Sleep-maintenance Insomnia
I can't get to sleep AND I can't stay asleep	→	Mixed Insomnia
Daytime (My poor sleep results in...)	Check (→)	
Fatigue or low energy	→	
Daytime sleepiness	→	Insomnia with daytime consequences
Mental impairments (e.g. attention, memory)	→	
Mood disturbance (e.g. irritability, feeling low)	→	
Poor performance (e.g. work, responsibilities)	→	
Problems with others (e.g. family, friends)	→	
Severity (These are problems for me...)	Check (→)	
Once or twice a week	→	Mild
Three or more nights a week	→	Severe
For less than three months	→	Acute
For more than three months	→	Persistent

Figure 15: Left panel: Case example of Charlotte's profile
Right panel: My insomnia profile

ASSESSING YOUR INSOMNIA PROBLEM

Night-time (My problem is that...)	Check (→)	
I can't get to sleep at the start of the night	→	Sleep-onset Insomnia
I can't stay asleep during the night	→	Sleep-maintenance Insomnia
I can't get to sleep AND I can't stay asleep	→	Mixed Insomnia
Daytime (My poor sleep results in...)	Check (→)	
Fatigue or low energy	→	Insomnia with daytime consequences
Daytime sleepiness	→	
Mental impairments (e.g. attention, memory)	→	
Mood disturbance (e.g. irritability, feeling low)	→	
Poor performance (e.g. work, responsibilities)	→	
Problems with others (e.g. family, friends)	→	
Severity (These are problems for me...)	Check (→)	
Once or twice a week	→	Mild
Three or more nights a week	→	Severe
For less than three months	→	Acute
For more than three months	→	Persistent

BOX 1: MY SLEEP PROFILE

I have a . . .

Your personal sleep history

Having thought so far about what your sleep is like at the moment, and where some of the problems lie, I want us now to go back in time a bit. Those of us who work in clinical practice talk about 'taking a history'. What we mean is finding out as much as we can about a problem, about how it shows itself day to day, and about its development over a period of time. In simple terms, the idea is to obtain an accurate picture. Here, of course, we are concerned with your *personal* sleep history.

Obviously, I cannot take your history, but I want you to imagine you are attending my clinic. So, I have provided you with a structure that I would use for your sleep history in Table 3. This is what is called a *semi-structured* approach because it guides you to general areas of content (left column) and to ask yourself 'starter' questions (middle column) to focus upon the issues of interest. In the right-hand column I have given you some further questions to answer to go into topics in more detail.

Is now a good time for you to work your way through your sleep history? Now where did you put that notebook?! You will find a notebook or an electronic document really helpful throughout the CBT programme, because writing things down does help us to think about them and to figure them out. In doing your history you may find you have to check out some information with other people – perhaps a partner can recall important times or dates or events, or a parent or brother or sister may remember further back when you were younger. Your notes are also going to be helpful when it comes to reminding you of key points in the programme, and of the decisions and plans you have made for your sleep. Oh, and before I leave the topic of notebooks, don't get too hung up on being neat and tidy! Your notebook is . . . for taking notes. It doesn't need to be a thing of beauty or a work of art. Use your notebook as a working document or a working file – if you really want to have a finished product at the end of the day, you can write that up later from your notes.

You can see in Table 3 that the sleep history begins with your sleep pattern, its quality and how it is affecting you. At this stage try to think of these matters fairly generally, because later I will be introducing the use of a sleep diary that will help you collect some of this information in a more systematic way. Next in Table 3 you will see you are moving on to consider how and when your insomnia developed over the years and how you used to sleep when you were

Table 3: Your personal sleep history

Content Area	Starter Question	Further Questions
Presentation of the sleep problem		
Pattern	*What is the pattern of your sleep on a typical night?*	*How long does it take you to fall asleep?* *How often do you wake up?* *How long are you awake for during the night?* *How much sleep do you get?* *How many nights each week are like this?*
Quality	*How do you feel about the quality of your sleep?*	*Is it refreshing?* *Is it enjoyable?* *Is it restless?* *How would you describe it in your own words?*
Daytime effects	*How does your night's sleep affect your day?*	*Do you feel tired?* *Do you feel sleepy?* *Do you have problems concentrating?* *Do you feel irritable?* *What do you think your insomnia does to your day?* *When are your worst times of the day?*
Impact on your life	*How does your insomnia affect your quality of life?*	*What consequences does insomnia have for you?* *What are you not able to do because of insomnia?* *How would things be different in your life if you overcame your insomnia?*

Development of the sleep problem	Do you remember how and when your poor sleep started?	What were the events and circumstances then? What were the important dates and times? How has your sleep changed over time? Has anything happened that has made it worse? Has anything happened that has made it better?
Lifetime history of the sleep problem	Did you used to be a good sleeper?	How did you sleep as a child? How did you sleep as a teenager? How did you sleep as a younger adult? Were there previous episodes of poor sleep? Dates and times? Did these past episodes resolve? If so, how?
Family history of sleep and sleep problems	Do other people in your family have problems sleeping?	Do either of your parents have sleep difficulties (now or in the past)? What about brothers and sisters? What about extended family, including grandparents? Does anyone have problems that are similar to your problems sleeping?
General health and medical history	Have you generally kept in good health?	Have you had any major illnesses? Have any health problems been persistent ones? Dates and times? Have there been any recent changes in your health?
History of psychological well-being	Are you the kind of person who usually copes well?	Have you had any psychological problems? Any problems with anxiety or depression, or with stress? Dates and times?
Current and previous treatments for insomnia	Are you taking anything to help you sleep?	What (if any) medicines are you taking now to help you sleep? What have you taken in the past? Dates and times? Are you taking anything you have bought over the counter? What sorts of things have you tried to do yourself to help you sleep? What have you found that has worked and hasn't worked?

younger. As I mentioned, some of this might need to be discussed a bit with other people who have useful information to share. Moving on again, spend a bit of time considering whether other people in your family have had sleep problems, and whether those are like your problem, or different from it. It's important next to take into account your general health and psychological well-being, and how such factors might be associated in some way with poor sleep. Finally, in Table 3 I have asked you to think through and note down things you have tried before to improve your sleep, for how long you tried them, and how well you think you tried them. This is important in itself to have as a record. It is also important because your past experience will have an effect upon your expectation of any future therapy (including the one in this book!).

Checking for other sleep problems

There is one other part of your sleep history that is important, although I have put it separately in another table for you. These are questions that refer to types of sleep problems other than insomnia (Table 4). The CBT methods that I will describe in this book are *only* for the treatment of insomnia, so it is important for you to consider the possibility that you may have a different type of problem instead, or as well. In clinical practice, I call this a *screening procedure*, because it is simply a way of identifying possible problems.

Turning then to Table 4, it is important that you consider whether or not you might screen positive for *any other type* of sleep disorder. Just proceed as you did with the first part of the sleep history. The left column lists the different types of sleep disorder, the middle column gives you a starter question, and the right-hand column asks you some follow-up questions. Keep a note of anything relevant in your notebook. To take the example of sleep-related breathing disorder (SBD), you will see that there is first a question about snoring. That is because most people with SBD snore. However, lots of people snore but do not have breathing pauses that affect the quality of their sleep. It is breathing pauses and daytime sleepiness that are particularly important here, because they raise the possibility of a disorder known as obstructive sleep apnoea. The questions on the right will help you to explore these details further.

If you think that you may have any of these other sleep problems, then you should read Chapter 16 in Part Four. I have added this chapter to give you advice on what to do, in addition to overcoming your insomnia. Of course, if you think that none of these screening questions is relevant to you, you can simply carry on to the next section.

Table 4: Screening for other disorders of sleep

Content Area	Starter Question	Further Questions
Screening for sleep disorders other than insomnia		
Sleep-related breathing disorder (SBD)	*Are you a heavy snorer?*	*Do you have interrupted breathing during your sleep?* *Does your partner say that you sometimes stop breathing?* *Do you wake up gasping for a breath?* *Are you excessively sleepy during the day?* *Do you fall asleep in the day without wanting to?*
Periodic limb movements in sleep (PLMS) and restless legs syndrome (RLS)	*Do your legs sometimes twitch or jerk or can't keep still?*	*Is it difficult to get to sleep because of muscle jerks?* *Do you wake from sleep with sudden jerky movements or feeling the need to move your legs?* *Do you have to get out of bed and pace around to get rid of these feelings?* *Are you excessively sleepy during the day?*
Circadian rhythm sleep disorders – delayed sleep phase syndrome (DSPS)	*Do you tend to sleep all right but at the 'wrong' time?*	*Can you sleep well enough but only if you stay up very late?* *Are you alert and not sleepy until a long while after normal bedtime?* *Are you sound asleep at normal waking time and can sleep on for hours?*

Circadian rhythm sleep disorders – advanced sleep phase syndrome (ASPS)	*Can you sleep well enough but only if you go to bed very early?* *Are you very sleepy if you try to stay up until normal bedtime?* *Do you wake very early, bright and alert and no longer sleepy?*
Parasomnias *Do you have unusual behaviours associated with your sleep?*	*Do you sleepwalk?* *Do you sleeptalk?* *Do you have confused behavioural episodes during the night?* *Do you have night terrors when you are very distressed but not properly awake?* *Do you grind your teeth at night?* *Do you sometimes act out your dreams? Do you have nightmares?*
Narcolepsy *Do you sometimes just fall asleep without warning?*	*Do you have sudden 'sleep attacks'?* *Is it impossible to resist falling asleep during the day?* *Do you have collapses and extreme muscle weakness triggered by emotion?* *Do you have hallucinations or odd sensations when you fall asleep or when you wake in the morning?* *Do you sometimes feel paralyzed and unable to move when you wake from your sleep?*

Using a sleep diary

Sometimes insomnia can be difficult to put into numbers. Ask yourself the question 'How long was I awake last night?' It's not just that it is hard to remember exactly. There is quite a challenge in adding up all the bits of time involved. Also, you may not quite think of your sleep in that way. You may reflect more generally on a 'good night' or a 'bad night', depending upon how you feel in the morning. This is because the *quality* of your sleep is just as important as its *quantity*.

Although it is not an easy task, I believe it is important for you to try to measure *both* your sleep pattern and your sleep quality as best as you can. This is where the sleep diary comes in. I have prepared a diary for you that leaves space for seven nights on one sheet (Figure 16). You should make an electronic version of this (or use the one available at www.colinespie.com) so that you can use it over and over while you follow the treatment programme. You will get better at filling in the diary with practice!

Your sleep diaries will help you to be more specific about where problems lie for you. For example, is it a difficulty getting to sleep, or a difficulty staying asleep, or is it both; and what nights are the worst? The diary will also help you look at your sleep across the week. You will be able to see any variability in sleep pattern or sleep quality from night to night, and to compare 'good nights' with 'bad nights'. Most importantly of all, the diary will also help you to assess changes in your sleep as you put the CBT programme into practice.

Week Beginning

Measuring the Pattern of Your Sleep

	Day 1	Day 2	Day 3	Day 4	Day 5	Day 6	Day 7
1. What time did you wake up this morning?							
2. What time did you rise from bed this morning?							
3. What time did you go to bed last night?							
4. What time did you put the light out?							
5. How long did it take you to fall asleep?							
6. How many times did you wake in the night?							
7. How long were you awake *during* the night?							
8. How long did you sleep together?							
9. How much alcohol did you have last night?							
10. How many sleeping pills did you take?							

Measuring the Quality of Your Sleep

1. How well rested do you feel this morning?

   0   1   2   3   4
not at all moderately very

2. Was your sleep of good quality?

   0   1   2   3   4
not at all moderately very

Figure 16: Your sleep diary

Have a detailed look now at Figure 16. You will see that the diary starts by asking you about your wake-up time and your rising time. These are the times when you finally woke up in the morning and when you finally got out of bed. Next you have to think back and note down your bedtime, and also when you put your light out the previous night. Then there are four questions about your sleep pattern – how long it took you to fall asleep, how many times you woke up in the night, how long in total these wakings lasted, and how long you think that you slept altogether. There is a bit of arithmetic involved! But hopefully you can make a reasonable estimate of all of these important dimensions of your sleep. Don't overthink it!

It is always a good idea to take note of anything that might have affected how you slept. You will see that I have put in questions about any alcohol or sleeping pills you took the night before. The pills section is easy – you can just put in the number you took, or the milligram (mg) dose if you prefer. For alcohol, I suggest you count in common 'units' where one small glass of wine, one standard measure (single) of spirits, and one half-pint or regular bottle of normal strength beer = 1 unit.

Finally, there are two questions on measuring the quality of your sleep. I have made this into a simple scale so you can just put in a number (0, 1, 2, 3 or 4) to represent how you feel about your sleep now that you have woken up. The higher the score, the better the quality of your sleep. After a while the numbers will begin to mean more to you!

Hopefully the diary is quite simple to understand. If you think it looks a bit complicated, I am sure that once you try it out over a few nights you will soon get the hang of it. I have made a few other suggestions in Box 2 that will help you to make the best use of your sleep diary. Read through these carefully.

BOX 2: SOME TIPS ON COMPLETING YOUR SLEEP DIARY

DO

- complete your diary within 1 hour of rising from bed
- write down times to the nearest 5 to 10 minutes if you can
- double-check your answers
- fill in every box
- keep your diary in a place you will find it each morning (e.g. next to your breakfast cereal box!)

DON'T

- clock-watch during the night
- worry about it! (it is just a record of your sleep)
- make up answers (it's OK to leave it blank if you forget!)

Recognising your baseline

Before you even start using the sleep diary, I would suggest that you have a think about what you expect your diary answers will look like. You might want to take a copy of the diary, mark it 'My Diary Estimate', and fill in just one column (any column) to represent what you think your sleep pattern and quality is like on a 'typical' night. You can then go ahead and start recording your sleep day by day using the diary and compare what you find after one week with your diary estimate. You can also have a think back to your sleep history and what you thought then about your sleep pattern.

Why am I suggesting using a diary? This is because, in my experience, people often learn quite a bit just from keeping a record. There may be things that confirm your expectations, and also things that are not what you expected at all! All of this is useful information when it comes to planning your new sleep schedule and adopting the right frame of mind to overcome insomnia.

I want you to *keep your diary from now on right through the treatment programme*. Let me tell you right now that you will find this a challenge! It is so easy to forget . . . and even a couple of minutes set aside to fill it in may seem like too much at the start of a busy day. Nevertheless, it is well worth the effort and it is very important. Have another look at the tips in Box 2, I hope they help.

In science, we talk of 'establishing a baseline'. This means that we try to establish what the problem we are trying to solve actually looks like. The information from your diary, along with your sleep condition indicator score (Figure 13) and the summary description of your problem (Box 1) give us detail and importantly give us data on the problem. When we have such data, we can then be more sure of whether or not we are making a difference through our intervention. Your sleep diary therefore is a record of your problem and a record of your progress in overcoming your insomnia using CBT.

Setting Your Goals

It is one thing to come to know what the problem looks like. It is another to decide what outcomes you are looking for as the solution! What are your goals in using this book? What are you trying to achieve through CBT? I want to think this one through carefully with you, because your success in overcoming your insomnia will be partly determined by your goals. This is an important statement, so let me repeat it:

> *Your success in overcoming your insomnia will be partly determined by your goals.*

If your goal is to sleep 8 hours every night, then by definition you would be unsuccessful if you achieved only 7½ hours, or if you did achieve 8 hours but only on some nights. It seems to me that when it comes to numbers, you are best to pitch at the most *achievable* figure that is *acceptable* to you. This is one way that the sleep condition indicator and the diary come in handy because you can find out what shape you are in at the start. As you go along, of course, you can always revise your goals. I think it is better to get encouragement by making improvements towards your (final) goal, by recognising progress you have made as compared with your baseline. I would advise you to set realistic goals at all times. If you have a handicap of 20 in golf, hoping to play off 10, would you rather be encouraged at achieving an interim goal of 15 or discouraged because you are only halfway there?

With sleep, though, as we know, it is not just numbers. What if your goal is 'just to get a decent night's sleep'? I have heard this so often . . . and no, it doesn't seem like too much to ask! However, the problem is that it is hard to know how you go about scoring this kind of goal. How do you define 'a decent night's sleep'? How do you know when you have achieved it? I think you need to find a way to make your goal *measurable*. In Table 5 I have given you a list of the categories of treatment goal that I commonly see at my clinics. Which of these, or which mixture of these, best describes the situation with your sleep?

Table 5: Different types of treatment goal

Common goals patients with insomnia want to achieve . . .	They say things like . . .
More sleep	'I'm simply not getting enough sleep. It feels like I hardly sleep at all and that's no good'
A more satisfying sleep	'I feel my sleep quality is really the problem . . . even when I do sleep, I never feel I've slept properly'
A more restorative sleep	'I want to be able to feel I can cope with the day . . . to feel rested and not tired all the time'
A more reliable sleep	'What sleep pattern? I don't have any pattern, that's the problem'
A more normal sleep	'I just want to get 7 or 8 hours . . . just like other people seem to manage'

You may feel that your first requirement is for *more sleep*. You feel that you are not getting enough of it. You may wish to fall asleep more quickly, to stay asleep without waking, or just to get a greater amount of sleep. Alternatively, you may feel that the sleep that you do get is not of acceptable quality and so you are seeking a *more satisfying sleep*. Here you want your sleep to be a nice sleep, an enjoyable experience.

Another possibility is that you are concerned mostly about the consequences of your sleep. You may feel, therefore, that you need a *more restorative sleep* to enable you to function properly in the daytime. On the other hand, if you feel your sleep pattern is out of control, you may be concerned about the inconsistency of your sleep. This is what I mean by talking of the goal of a *more reliable* sleep, a pattern you can rely upon to be OK. Finally, you might think in terms of wanting to have a *normal* sleep. This might be a goal of sleeping in the way that other people seem to sleep, or in the way you yourself were able to sleep in the past.

The message is to know your problem, but also to know your goals. Write down your goals in your notebook now . . . but, because your goals in overcoming insomnia need to be considered carefully, I strongly recommend that you are always prepared to come back to these key questions:

- Is my sleep goal *achievable*? Am I setting the bar too high? (remember that you can come back and re-set the goals a step at a time)
- Is the sleep goal that is achievable *acceptable* to me? Does it motivate me? Will I see it as progress?
- Is my achievable and acceptable sleep goal *measurable*? How will I know when I have reached the goal?

Are you ready?

The final thing I want you to assess before we move on is your *motivation* for CBT. Don't be offended! It's not that

I doubt your commitment to try to improve your sleep. I know that you are likely to have tried loads of things before. In fact, that is one of the reasons I mention motivation. It can be hard to try again after many disappointments, and perhaps you have limited confidence that anything will ever work.

It is particularly important that I ask the question 'are you ready?' with a CBT programme, because CBT can be very demanding of you. I tell you, even to keep up with those diaries will at times feel tiresome! You are also going to face some tough decisions about your sleep and about your beliefs and attitudes concerning your sleep. There will be things to do . . . and things to give up.

Then again, changes take time so please be gentle with yourself if you don't find improvements occurring as quickly as you would like. They say that 'old habits die hard' and you will need to coax new habits to develop! Keeping motivated is the key to feeling encouraged and to achieving permanent improvements in your sleep pattern.

The diagram in Figure 17 shows us the process of changing a situation. Where are you on this wheel at the moment? First you have to consider whether you are interested in addressing your sleep problem at this particular point in time. That's what I mean by using the words 'thinking about changing'. As you can see, considering whether or not CBT might be for you comes before the second step, which is actively deciding that you want to follow the course. Bear in mind that some practical obstacles may delay you if you don't deal with them just now. It's worth spending a bit of time writing down what you think might help and what you think might hinder you.

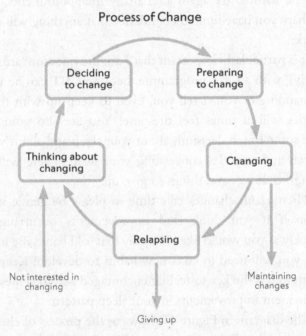

Process of Change

Figure 17: Considering your motivational state

If all is set fair to progress from the thinking and deciding stage, then what is the next step? The third stage is about making all the necessary preparations to get started in a practical sense. So far, that will have involved reading Part One of this book, working on your sleep history, photocopying your sleep diary, and so on. If you progressed beyond that to implementing 'changing' at the fourth step then you will have done things like recording your sleep estimates, keeping your diary, and you will have carefully thought through and written down your sleep goals.

I want you to come back to this diagram as you implement elements of CBT during the programme and ask yourself the question, 'Where am I on this wheel at the moment?' Your motivation to follow CBT may come and go; that is to be expected. Some parts of the course are challenging, so do expect ups and downs. Try to correct your course towards positive actions if things have slipped. You will see in Figure 17 that mention is made of relapsing. *Relapses* are times when you experience a strong feeling of disappointment either with the programme, because you hoped it would have worked better or more quickly; or with yourself, because you felt unable to follow a part of the programme or you forgot to do it. You may find that your sleep improves but then gets worse (relapses) again. These are all examples of times you may think that there is no point in continuing. Please don't let such relapses discourage you. The best thing to do is to get back to the CBT course and try again.

I want to reassure you that I am telling you this because it is quite normal for the process of sleep change to be an uneven path. Try to think of that as normal and you will find it much easier to deal with. Remember too that you have had this insomnia for a while. You may need to work hard to overcome it. Let me also tell you, though, that you may never have had a better chance of sorting out your sleep problems than this CBT programme! Remember it is an evidence-based approach, which means it has worked for many, many others who have seen it through. As you can see from Figure 17, your goal is to maintain all the changes that you are able to put into practice so that your new, good sleep pattern becomes permanent.

PART THREE

OVERCOMING YOUR INSOMNIA AND BECOMING A GOOD SLEEPER

Introduction to
Part Three

This is probably the part you have been waiting for, and perhaps the place you skipped to right from the start!? It's time to begin to put your CBT treatment plan in place and to help you overcome your insomnia. The background on sleep and on insomnia in Part One, and the assessment of your own sleep in Part Two should have provided you with a better understanding of your problems.

Indeed, think of where we are right now a bit like this. Supposing you had actually been attending my Sleep Clinic. So far, I would have been asking you questions, and listening to your answers; trying to understand your problems, your needs and your goals. I would have been explaining about sleep and insomnia along the way to help your understanding. Now that we know what kind of shape your sleep is in, we have got to the point where I can explain more about how I might be able to assist. Usually that is the question that people ask out loud, or at least have in their minds, at this juncture: *'do you think you can help me?'*

If you have a chronic insomnia disorder, I would then say 'yes' to that question and would explain more about what CBT is, and why it is the best choice of treatment for you. If you then decided that is what you want to pursue, we would work together to design your personal treatment plan. I'm going to use Part Three of the book now, to work with you in exactly these ways. Let's get going!

BOX 3: REASONS TO TRUST CBT AS THE BEST TREATMENT FOR CHRONIC INSOMNIA DISORDER

✓ CBT is the most suitable treatment because insomnia is a psycho-physiological disorder
✓ CBT has been rigorously tested and has the best clinical evidence to treat insomnia
✓ CBT for insomnia has many effective elements and can be easily personalised for your needs

---

7

Why CBT?

At several points already I have introduced CBT and emphasised that it is the recommended treatment of choice for insomnia. Now I want to go into a little more detail about what CBT is and, importantly, why it is the best option for treating chronic insomnia. In Box 3 I have listed the three main reasons why you should trust CBT to help you overcome your insomnia. Let's look at each of these reasons in turn.

CBT is the treatment best suited for insomnia

CBT is the most suitable treatment for insomnia, because insomnia is a psycho-physiological disorder. That's a bit of a mouthful, isn't it! What do I mean by 'psycho-physiological'?

I mean that when you have insomnia you struggle to sleep because of your racing mind, your difficulties relaxing and the challenges you have in getting normal sleep into a pattern that just flows naturally from night to night. Sleep becomes a big psychological issue, and you are aware of the self-defeating aspects of so much wanting to sleep, yet at the same time the sleeplessness and difficulties getting to sleep and staying asleep are very real. From a physiological point of view, you are too alert, and too aroused to sleep. It really has become a vicious cycle.

CBT is ideal to address these problems because the 'C' in CBT refers to those cognitive and emotional aspects, providing you with techniques that combat your mental alertness, worries in bed, and your racing mind; and the 'B' in CBT helps you re-discover and re-establish your natural sleep pattern, based on your personal sleep needs, and to get back into a proper sleep routine. Importantly, CBT clears the flightpath for the return of the dove and allows sleep to work in harmony with your body clock or circadian rhythm. You see, your sleep drive and your body clock aren't fundamentally broken. You just need CBT to re-engage automatic and natural good sleep, so your dove can stay.

CBT has the best evidence for treating insomnia

None of what I was saying above would matter if CBT didn't actually work. There's no point in having a key that fits if it cannot unlock the door!

All evidence summaries and all clinical guidelines around the world endorse CBT as having the best evidence for treating chronic insomnia both safely and effectively. Moreover, this is true for men and women of all ages, even dare I say including 'older' adults! It is also true whether or not you have another health problem, be it physical or mental, or indeed another sleep disorder. The guidelines are that chronic insomnia disorder should be treated, whenever it presents, even if other medical conditions are being treated at the same time. Of course, CBT does not involve taking medication so using CBT is less of a concern than taking drugs might be, especially if you have a comorbid condition. CBT for insomnia is clinically effective in around 70 per cent of people, even where the insomnia is very long-standing, and most people who do not make a full response still find CBT helpful.

As with all treatments for any condition, including insomnia disorder, it is always advisable to speak to your physician, clinical psychologist, or other health care provider first (depending upon whoever may be involved in your care). This is especially true if you remain concerned about any aspect of your health, but they will most likely know about CBT and will be reassured that CBT for insomnia disorder is the recommended treatment of first choice in clinical guidelines.

I should also mention that the CBT programme for insomnia that I have provided you with in this book has been part of the literature that led to these guidelines being developed. I have published scores of clinical studies and clinical trials on CBT since the late 1980s. I would not be writing this book if I was not confident of two things. First, that CBT works; and second that the CBT approach that I am providing you with works.

CBT has the most resources for treating insomnia

I want to let you into what seems to me to be like a well-kept secret. CBT is not a treatment. Let me say that again with the important emphasis: *CBT is not **a** treatment*.

People often talk about CBT as if it were a thing, like 'I tried CBT'. But my reaction to this would be 'what did you try?' Because to me when you say 'I tried CBT', I have little idea what was involved. If you were to say, 'I tried melatonin', or 'I tried Ambien', then that would be a bit more straightforward. I might just want to know 'what dose, how often and for how long': because drugs are more like 'things' to try.

I am saying that CBT is not *a* therapy but a *system of therapies*. You might think of it like this. Using a drug solution, or as we might call it, 'pharmacotherapy', tells us what kind of thing you tried; as in you took a pill; you took medication. However, it doesn't tell us what specific drug you took. Likewise, CBT is the family name, not the actual treatment name, and the good news is that CBT has many effective treatments in the family, and so CBT can be personalised for your needs. You may find as you work your way through this book that you major on just one element of CBT and that is enough, or you may find you use several, or all the things I suggest. This is where CBT is very versatile, and truly a substantial resource to help so many people with insomnia.

Cognitive Behavioural Therapeutics (CBTx)

So, let me introduce you to a new concept here that I hope will be useful. I am more and more using the term CBTx rather than CBT to highlight the fact that CBT is a therapeutic system, and that we can look within this resource system to find the best treatment to start with, and how to follow on when adding another treatment element.

This is a big change in this second edition of the book from the first edition. Back then I presented the book as a series of weekly sessions that you should do in order. This was because that was the way we treated most insomnia in those days; and you can still do it that way if you want to now. However, now we are using a more *personalised behavioural medicine* approach to devise your personal treatment plan. That is to find the best starting point for you, based upon your particular insomnia problem, and upon your own preferences about where to start.

The CBTx method also helps you to make sure that you get the most out of a given treatment technique. That you can if you like 'digest' it and get it into your system before adding more and more content. It also means that you may not have to do absolutely everything in the book to get a clinically meaningful improvement in your sleep. In the next chapter I will explain how this is all going to work.

Table 6: Developing your personal CBTx treatment plan

CBTx therapeutic domain	How it helps	Power	Difficulty	Location
Cognitive	Dealing with your racing mind	***	***	Chapter 9
Behavioural	Establishing your new sleep pattern	*****	****	Chapter 10
Relaxation	Reducing your arousal	**	**	Chapter 11
Support domain	How it helps	Power	Difficulty	Location
Lifestyle	Improving your sleep hygiene	*	*	Chapter 12
Education	Improving your sleep knowledge	*	*	Chapter 13

8

Developing Your Personal Treatment Plan

Have a close look at Table 6. It is going to be a central navigational aid for you to help you plan your personalised CBTx journey.

In the far left column, you will see that I have listed five domains. Three of these are therapeutics and two are support domains. In the second column I have noted what that treatment component mainly addresses. I say 'mainly' because there is a degree of cross-over. Then further to the right, I have given you an indication of how strong a treatment effect might be associated with each domain. I have called this 'power', as in how powerful it usually is to address insomnia problems. You need to consider this as an average though, because some treatment elements are stronger for some people. You also need to bear in mind that they all have some effect. The next column to the right is labelled 'difficulty', meaning how challenging I think it is to implement the techniques in that area – if you like, how much it requires of you. Then finally, in the column furthest to the right, you are directed to where you can find all the details on the treatments themselves. At this point though, let me give you a brief summary of each domain area.

Cognitive therapeutics

Techniques in this area are primarily directed at mental events and experiences that might be keeping you awake. Cognitive techniques therefore address the racing mind as the enemy of sleep, whether those thoughts are focused on past, present or future events; on rehearsing – replaying – the day that has just gone and planning the day ahead; on worries, fears, frustrations or sadness; trivial or random thoughts; or on sleep and sleeplessness itself. The general theme is an active mind and not being able to shut it down mentally and emotionally. This may all sound very familiar, and indeed the thing that people with insomnia most commonly believe is responsible for being unable to sleep is an overactive mind.

Cognitive therapeutic methods are effective, as you can see in the Table 6 power rating. They are not the most powerful but are strong as an overall effect. The limiting factor to their effectiveness is that they do not directly address your sleep pattern, and if your sleep efficiency is poor, cognitive therapeutics alone may not enable you to sleep through the night.

Behavioural therapeutics

These techniques help to establish a regular sleep rhythm

from night to night and are designed to eliminate wakefulness from your bedtime experience. Behavioural therapeutics essentially tell you what to do and when, and how to do it; rather than how to think differently. Examples include establishing a regular time to retire to bed and to rise in the morning, knowing what to do when you are lying awake at night, and strengthening the automatic connection between being in bed and sleeping. The approach is very practical, first of all focusing on discovering your personal sleep requirement and how to get from where you are now to where you want to be.

I, along with most experts in insomnia across the world, regard behavioural therapeutics as the most effective, especially if you have a sleep efficiency below 80 per cent. They do not directly address the racing mind, but because you quite quickly sleep better they have the reassuring effect that sleep is becoming stronger. The behavioural techniques are the hardest to implement. They are quite demanding at first because they involve changing your sleep pattern, usually spending less time in bed initially so that sleep drive strengthens.

Relaxation therapeutics

As you can see in Table 6, relaxation methods, of which there are many, are helpful if you feel the need to relax and to reduce your level of arousal. It's hard to fall asleep if you are not relaxed and similarly hard to get back to sleep. Some people say that they are too 'wound up' to sleep. They experience a kind of sleep stress response where muscle tension or other physical symptoms such as restlessness in bed, palpitations, hearing their heartbeat, and getting hot and sweaty, prevent them from sleeping well. Quite often people who feel like this are just not very relaxed people, so relaxation therapeutics can be useful to them more generally.

Relaxation methods are usually liked by people who use them, and they are somewhat easier to put into practice than cognitive or behavioural methods. However, they are not as powerful in helping you overcome insomnia. Although being relaxed helps you to be better prepared for bed and for sleep, it has a lesser effect on insomnia as a disorder.

Lifestyle support

As you can see, Table 6 also includes two *support domains* that may be helpful as you address the three main therapeutic areas. The first of these relates broadly to your lifestyle and to elements of what is commonly known as *sleep hygiene*. Things like the comfort and suitability of your bedroom environment and your health habits are what I have in mind. In itself, sleep hygiene intervention is not an effective treatment for insomnia. This is why I have given it a low power rating. On the other hand, there may be elements that are easily addressed and if you feel that any of them is relevant, then you should consider including them in your treatment plan.

Education support

The point I would make about sleep education is that although growing your knowledge and understanding is always a good thing; knowing something and acting upon it are very different challenges. Part One, for example, contains a lot of information, and I would encourage you to read and re-read it, but more important is to use that knowledge to inform and motivate your actions in relation to cognitive, behavioural and relaxation therapeutics. Knowledge will give you the why, the therapeutics give you the what and the how. For example, because you understand how sleep is regulated, behavioural intervention makes more sense; and because you have information about the brain's role in emotion regulation, cognitive approaches to the racing mind seem like a good fit.

Where to start?

Your instinct

A glance at Table 6, supported by my comments above on each domain, may give you an instinct about what chapter to navigate to first of all to begin your treatment course. It's up to you to choose. Don't worry, it's not a crucial decision; you can't get it terribly wrong!

My thinking in giving you options is that this is what we would discuss if you were at my Sleep Clinic. We would talk through the possibilities and I would give you my advice to help you to choose. I've already been doing so by saying this is what this works for, this is how effective this is, this one is more or less challenging and so on. Giving you options, however, is also about giving you more control. Not control over sleep itself, because no-one really has, or needs, that; but control over the treatment process. I believe this will help you to take more responsibility for finding a solution and for putting it into practice. It will also give you greater confidence that *you* have managed to overcome your insomnia problem, with help and guidance. It's not a magic bullet from me!

Your data

Remember too that you already have data to help you decide where to start. You know yourself and what 'rings true' from Table 6, but you also have data from what you have been doing so far, like completing the sleep condition indicator and your sleep diary. You can work out, for example, what your sleep efficiency is. You can also gather more data if you need to before beginning CBT.

You will also find that, at the beginning of each of the therapeutics chapters, I have provided you with further ways to evaluate whether or not this is a good starting point. For example, I will help you figure out what your sleep efficiency is, so that you can see if behavioural therapeutics might help. I will help you consider what type of racing mind you suffer from most, so you can select from amongst a range of cognitive therapeutics the ones that may be most helpful. I will help you also to consider what relaxation strategy would be best for your situation. In other words, in each of the main therapies chapters there is further navigational support available, and we will use your own data to assist there.

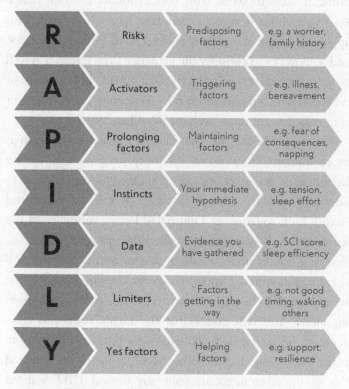

Figure 18: RAPIDLY developing a formulation (shared understanding) of your insomnia problem and how to treat it

Our formulation

You may have noticed that I have switched quite deliberately in this heading to the word 'our'. Why is that? Why *our formulation*? 'Formulation' is a term that is used in clinical psychology to refer to a shared understanding of what the problem is, how it may have developed, and what keeps it going. I want to work with you to follow the best *clinical hypotheses* about how your insomnia might be solved. This approach incorporates your instinct, and your preferences, and it allows us to consider the evidence from research as well as your own data, and to formulate a plan, not only about where to start but also about how to sequence the treatment elements that are most likely to be of benefit to you.

Now admittedly, this shared or *collaborative* approach is more difficult, because we can only imagine that we are in the same room at my Sleep Clinic. Nevertheless, let's continue with the mental picture that you are there; and have a look together at Figure 18. I have summarised the formulation. It is sometimes called the *case conceptualisation*; that is, a way of understanding your insomnia problem. All these jargon words, I know! However, the good news is that it only needs to be a quick way to get to a *good enough working model*. You will notice that the formulation also takes account of anticipated challenges to putting solutions in place – they might even be barriers that get in the way and that you need to negotiate your way around. CBT is about implementing effective treatment elements, whilst also taking account of how we problem solve around obstacles to putting our best intentions into practice. As you can see, it's not just about obstacles or challenges though; a formulation also takes into account the strengths that you have available to you.

Let's do it RAPIDLY

I'm not so much referring to speed here, but to following a process for making sure that we get a good formulation of your problems. Have an in-depth look at Figure 18 where you'll see that I have used what's called a 'mnemonic' – the word 'RAPIDLY' as a way of summarising what we need to take into account in devising a formulation.

You may recall from Figure 9 in Part One that I explained about how insomnia developed. Then I spoke about pre-disposing, precipitating and perpetuating factors. I have simplified the language here in Figure 18 to risk, activate and prolong factors; the RAP in RAPIDLY!

Have a think about what might have put you at *risk* (R) for developing insomnia. Something that made you more vulnerable to being a poor sleeper or to waking up. Remember this risk factor isn't enough in its own right to cause insomnia to happen; it just means that it increases the chances that you might develop it, or, to put it another way, it makes you more vulnerable. I've given examples in Figure 18. Were you a very light sleeper as a child? Are you prone to worry? A night owl? A risk factor doesn't need to be something that has always been there. It could be more recent, it could be a change in life circumstances, and it could be a positive thing, like being very organised and liking to be in control. The point is that there was some fertile ground for the seeds of insomnia to grow, and there may have been more than one risk factor.

Now think about anything that has in your experience activated symptoms of insomnia, even though this may have been quite temporary. This activate phase is about triggers that have pushed you into sleeplessness. There may be examples of *activators* (A) that are more substantial, like losing your job, children moving away from home, worry about a test result; or examples of more fleeting stresses like an awkward conversation, misplacing something and not being able to find it, or a stressful social occasion coming up. The point here is that symptoms of insomnia at such times are more likely to become hard to manage if there is an underlying greater vulnerability to insomnia. Can you see how risk and activation might interact with one another?

Often people really struggle to understand the *prolong* phase (P). They say to me at the Sleep Clinic, *'I have my health, and a great family, I went through a difficult spell back [whenever], but now I really don't have anything to worry about. Why on earth can't I sleep? I don't have any good reason for having insomnia.'* This is a great example of the prolong phase because, in this case, we have a vicious circle established where stress about sleep and sleeplessness itself is the factor that is maintaining the insomnia. So, what do you think prolongs your insomnia? Do you get caught up in it all? Are you over-thinking it? Do you feel you waken up as soon as you go to bed and your head hits the pillow? Usually, the factors that prolong insomnia are not the ones that activate it. Anyone can have a brief spell of poor sleep when they are stressed, but it normally goes away. What keeps your insomnia going?

Just a little while ago we spoke about the I for *instinct,* and the D for *data.* You will see them in Figure 18. As we think about the formulation of your sleep problem we are generating and testing hypotheses, theories and ideas about why you are having these problems with your sleep. I really encourage you to listen to your instincts. What do you think? What about asking other people whom you trust and test your hypothesis about how risk, activate and prolong factors interact in your case? You should keep the best hypotheses and discard ones that don't appear to be true. It's like detective work to see if there is evidence for your instinct.

Importantly, go in search of data to test your hypotheses – ask yourself the question 'is there evidence that . . .', ask other people what they think, look at the data in your sleep diary. Think about what sources of information there might be to help you to answer your questions, and gather more data. I always encourage my patients to look to the facts and not just to your feelings. So, it's also important to evaluate whatever information you gather. It's not that how we feel is unimportant. Emotions matter, as do hunches and instincts, as I have been saying. But it is a really useful discipline, and one that is central to CBT, to ask yourself where are the data on this?

Let's take stock of where we are so far with our formulation. Steadily now, if not rapidly (!), we are formulating your problem. It's always good to understand, to have an explanation for something that's been a problem, and a puzzling problem perhaps. But it's about more than that, it's also about where the explanation leads us in terms of planning a treatment. It's like an 'if–then' relationship. For example, if it's true that I have got into the habit of being very tense in bed, then I need a treatment that helps me be less tense in bed. Relaxation therapeutics help us to reduce our arousal, cognitive therapeutics to deal with our minds, and behavioural therapeutics to establish good sleep patterns. These are all 'if–thens'. Look again at Table 6. Is our formulation helping you to decide where to start your treatment plan?

As you think towards a particular starting point, I would strongly encourage you to consider the last part of the RAPIDLY approach; that is the LY. What is going to get in the way of you starting your therapy? What might be the *limiters* (L), the obstacles to implementing changes in your routines. We will think more about these within each of the treatment sections to come, but don't be naïve. It really pays to imagine yourself following your CBT programme and trying to generate all the possible barriers, so that you can overcome them of course. If the limiting factors are the downside, the *yes factors* (Y) are the upside. Try to think about what and who might help, and how. It's great if you are a resourceful and committed person, and that you are saying 'yes' to the time being right to start your CBT now, but we all need encouragement and support at times. Overcoming insomnia is not always easy. I guess if it were you wouldn't be needing this book!

I want you to have a go at writing down your own formulation in your notebook, now that we have been through the RAPIDLY process. Remember that what we need is a *good enough working model*. You can add or change things as we go through, as you get new insights. For example, if you have a hypothesis that managing your thinking differently will reduce your worry about sleep and so you will sleep better; and that hypothesis is found to be true from experience using cognitive therapeutics then all well and good. It helps confirm your theory. But if on the other hand you are still stuck with the problem despite working on a particular cognitive approach then it is good to *re-formulate*, and possibly go in a different direction where perhaps a different cognitive technique might be a better 'if–then' than the one you were using; or you may figure out that a behavioural or relaxation approach now seems to make more sense. You can also blend effective strategies because more than one explanation may be true, and elements of your formulation may interact.

To help you complete your formulation, I have given you the example of Will's formulation in Box 4. Read it through. Hopefully it is fairly self-explanatory, and will help you to draft out your own.

BOX 4: WILL'S *GOOD ENOUGH EXPLANATION* FOR HAVING CHRONIC INSOMNIA, USING THE RAPIDLY FORMULATION MODEL

Will (aged 42) has been thinking through why he has insomnia. He is considering how it may have developed, what keeps it going now, and importantly what he might do about it, and how. He's bearing in mind factors that he thinks might help

---

him overcome his insomnia, and barriers that might get in the way. Listen to what he told me:

I'm thinking that I've never really been a good sleeper. Even my mum tells me I woke at the drop of a hat as a baby. I also was a bit poorly during secondary school and woke up quite a bit with stomach cramps. I'm thinking that these might be RISK factors as to why I would be more vulnerable to developing insomnia in the first place.

But I wouldn't say I really had any sleep problems as such until I left university and started my first job. I had a lot on my mind, and a lot of work to do. In the first few weeks I struggled to get to sleep and woke up quite a bit, but put it down to normal stress really, and it probably was. So, this for me was possibly what triggered my insomnia back then; an ACTIVATOR. Yes, I do think I react to stress at times.

I never really thought about it too much, as I said, but I remember I began to think about sleep really for the first time. That I had to make sure that I would get enough sleep, otherwise I wouldn't manage during the day. I found myself beginning to go to bed earlier and then if I couldn't sleep getting angry about it. That only made it worse. This was for sure the PROLONG stage when my insomnia became a problem, like with a life of its own.

My insomnia has come and gone over the years. Well, never really quite gone. It's always there in the background. I've kinda got used to it, although the last 3 years have been really bad. I've partly got into the habit of organising my life around sleep because worrying about sleep is something I do even during the day. I've turned down opportunities to take on more responsibility in case I failed. My INSTINCT is that my problem with sleep is over-thinking it all the time.

Since coming to the Sleep Clinic I've been completing the measures you gave me. I was happy that the sleep condition indicator showed me to be a very poor sleeper. I felt it vindicated my experience! Not too many people understand what it feels like to have insomnia. The diary has been really helpful, and I discovered from my DATA that my sleep efficiency is down at 72 per cent. I'm thinking now that the cognitive therapeutics piece seems very relevant to me, but that I'll also need to look into the behavioural part of the programme because of my poor sleep efficiency.

I'd never really thought before that I would have choices about what to do and that someone would help me weigh them up. I thought the doctor would like just say 'do this' or 'do that'. So when I think of putting some CBT into practice, I realise that there are some LIMITERS for me; or at least they are obstacles in my head. The main one right now is how I could do a challenging programme like sorting out my sleep pattern. We have a young baby at home and I feel I need to grab any sleep I can get and not just choose when I want to go to bed and get up. It feels a bit selfish and I'm not sure my wife would appreciate that.

On the other hand, we have a very good relationship, and it was she who told me to go and get some help in the first

> *place! I guess I could discuss it with her? It's not as if it's a secret at home and I would be in a much better place to help out and be a good partner if I didn't have this insomnia thing on my back all the time. I guess this is what you mean by a YES factor. I would have support, I think. Besides, I'm not the kind of person who likes to be beaten by things. Maybe this is one of the reasons that I've put off getting help for so long – I wouldn't want to find that its unsolvable!*

Well done so far! One more thing before we move on to the therapeutics chapters.

Your commitment

I'm saying this now because it is true regardless of your treatment journey or your treatment combination. You need to make a commitment if you want CBT to work; and, related to that, you need to put therapy into regular practice if it's going to help you overcome insomnia. In Table 6 I gave you the impression that some parts of therapy take more effort than others. Whereas this is true, it is also true that I need you to be committed to whatever we work on together. If I am to help you that is.

My CBT programme is based on many years of careful clinical and research work, conducted in general medical practice settings as well as specialised settings. It is a programme for people like you with severe and enduring insomnia, and my aim is to pass on to you a clinically proven and effective treatment. As you know, you are best to think of this as if you are attending my Sleep Clinic for a course of treatment. Instead of me acting as your therapist, the book, I hope, will do it instead! Certainly, I have written it for you with this in mind, and this is my commitment to you.

Just as I would if we were in the same room, I am asking for a commitment in return. Not for my sake, but for yours. Because otherwise the whole exercise is rather pointless. It does happen in clinical practice, believe me, and it is not intentional, but people show up but do relatively little else. People try, really try, to work on things, and they intend to follow through on actions and plans. The problem is, we are all full of good intentions; and it is actually quite hard to make changes, even when we want and need them. I genuinely understand this, as I hope you'll see as we go through the therapy options. This is why the L and the Y are part of the formulation – know the limitations and the strengths that you have and that are in your situation. Know them not only by instinct but by evidence. Are you, for example, still keeping your sleep diary?

When I raise the subject of commitment people sometimes ask how much they have to do to get a good treatment response. This is a very fair question, and I love it when they ask that. It implies to me a recognition of the truth that we are all imperfect, but at the same time a willingness to hold themselves accountable. Now, if I were giving you pills that question (of what do I need to do) would be easily answered e.g., take those pills as prescribed every night for the duration of the prescription. But you know it's really exactly the same with CBT, you need to take the behavioural medicine. In CBT that means putting things into practice on a day-to-day – well, night-to-night – basis. The dose of CBT is the doing of it. I say this to my patients *'dose equals implementation'*. There's no point having the solution and not implementing it; and it won't work if you don't do it.

So, let me be clear, this is not a reading exercise. The book is more like a manual – a *what* to do, *how* to do it, *when* to do it, kind of book. Hopefully, it will also be clear from your formulation *why* you are doing what you are doing. Do try to give your reading and preparation for CBT some priority time so that you can make the most of the advice I can give you. If you were really coming along to see me, you would be setting aside time. Plus, you would have the 'homework' aspect to it, too, because you would be putting into practice what we had agreed. You need to follow this same kind of discipline here if you want to get the most benefit from the book. Have a think now about when you can set aside time each week to concentrate on the material you need to cover.

I think of your task as a cycle of reading, understanding, applying and reviewing . . . as you go along. It's good to go back over things again and again to make sure that you really understand. As you put things into practice you will understand even better. By reviewing how things are going with your sleep pattern, you will be giving yourself feedback on your success in applying what you have learned and will have the opportunity to check if you are following each part of the CBT programme correctly. On the next read-through, perhaps you will pick up on something else. I'm sure you get what I mean – the bottom line is that this course requires quite a bit from you. Keep going round that cycle!

A final, final word. People sometimes ask what is the secret ingredient of CBT? Why does it work for so many people who have such engrained insomnia problems? I'll let you into that secret, and I've already mentioned it. CBT unlocks sleep to work for you. The secret ingredient is the power of your natural sleep-wake rhythm. CBT gets sleep back into shape and occurring naturally, exactly like it does for the good sleeper.

Let the dove return – it wants to sit there!

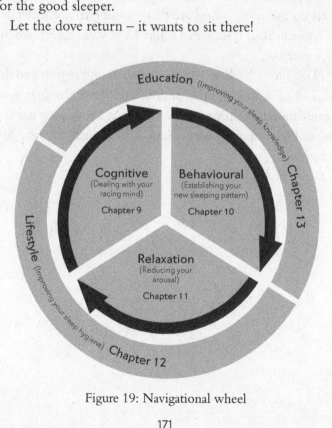

Figure 19: Navigational wheel

Navigating to your CBT starting point

OK, so now it's over to you to decide the starting point for your CBTx journey! You can begin with the cognitive (Chapter 9) *or* the behavioural (Chapter 10) *or* the relaxation therapeutics (Chapter 11) – whichever you think is best for you. I have provided you with a navigational wheel (Figure 19) so you can quickly get to the content of each chapter. Then you can work through the other parts of the inner therapy wheel. The sleep knowledge and sleep hygiene parts on the outer wheel are there to support your therapy, so you can read Chapters 12 and 13 at your leisure whenever you like.

Have a look back at Table 6 to refresh on the pros and the cons of each therapeutics option; and think through your formulation to help you make a decision about your starting point. Please don't worry about it too much though. Just get going!

Good luck!

9

Dealing With Your Racing Mind – Cognitive Therapeutics

Introduction

Welcome to the chapter on the 'C' from CBT! Yes, that's right, the cognitive part, where we will be looking at the mental events and experiences that might be keeping you awake. If you have started here, it's probably because the racing mind is a major issue for you. But even if you have been working on some other chapter first, I'm sure that this is going to be very relevant.

So often people have said to me that their main problem is not being able to empty their mind . . . not being able to stop their thoughts from racing. Sometimes they say that they feel physically exhausted, but they just cannot seem to switch off mentally. Indeed, research studies have shown that people with insomnia are actually more aware of *mental* symptoms of arousal than they are of bodily (physiological) symptoms. That's one of the reasons why I wouldn't be surprised if you have headed straight here. I am going to take you through the strategies that we teach our patients to deal with thoughts and worries that interfere with sleep. I will also help you to identify the types of thought problems you are having – you may be having more than one – and find the best solution for you.

The purpose of cognitive therapeutics for insomnia then is *to learn ways of overcoming the mental alertness, repetitive thoughts and anxieties that interfere with your sleep.* Let's get going with that!

Knowing the enemy

Research has shown that people with insomnia complain a lot about a highly active mind in bed. They may or may not be the kind of people who have an overactive mind in the daytime, too. Some people seem to get into the habit of using their time in bed as a time to think things through. Maybe they lead busy daytime lives and just run out of thinking time. Others find that it is impossible to keep their minds empty when it is quiet and they can't sleep, and then they get preoccupied with their own thoughts – however important or trivial the thoughts may be. This busy and racing mind is the 'enemy of sleep'.

First of all, let's consider the kinds of things that you think about when you are in bed and unable to get to sleep. There are several types of thoughts that are common. They are summarised in Figure 20. I want you to consider each of these to see if they ring a bell. You can then try to match up my solution to that thought problem, and go straight there for help, or you can use several or all of the cognitive strategies to fight off your racing mind.

As you will see, some of the 'fight' is quite subtle, it's getting prepared and being on the front foot, outsmarting and even ignoring the enemy, not over-reacting, certainly not being bullied, and figuring out truth from fiction.

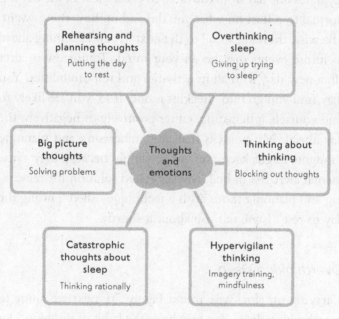

Figure 20: Why our minds might not turn off

Let me start by explaining each of the six thought problems, the reasons why our minds might not turn off, and then we will go through suggested solutions to each problem.

Rehearsing and planning thoughts

As the name suggests, this is when you think back over the day or recent events, or when you look ahead to things that are about to come up. Replaying the day's events at the end of the day is in some ways quite a natural thing to do. Perhaps it is even enjoyable at times! It just so happens that the night separates one day from the next, so at the close of the day it is normal to reflect on what you did and on how things went. Likewise, thinking ahead to the next day and planning ahead to future events may be on your mind. Tomorrow is, after all, a new day, with all its activities and responsibilities. You may find you go into checklist mode. If so, you are likely to find yourself anticipating, either positively or negatively, the day ahead. My point is that your rehearsing and planning thoughts might keep you awake simply because they cause mental alertness in bed. My suggested solution for rehearsing and planning thoughts is a technique called 'putting the day to rest'. I will tell you about it shortly.

Overthinking sleep

Carrying on clockwise round Figure 20, next we come to overthinking sleep. You may be in the habit of thinking a lot about sleep when you are in bed, or more likely, thinking a lot about the fact that you're *not* sleeping! When people have persistent insomnia, difficulty getting to sleep or difficulty getting back to sleep seems to become part of a vicious circle: I want to sleep – I can't sleep – I can't stop thinking about how to get to sleep – so I'm keeping myself awake

– and wanting to sleep even more. When sleep doesn't come quickly or naturally you may well find that you become preoccupied with your sleep and your sleeplessness. These kinds of thoughts often lead us to try too hard to get to sleep, and to be desperate to find a solution. Maybe thoughts that are very focused on sleep is a familiar part of your racing mind? As you will see my solution is perhaps a surprising one – to give up trying to sleep! I will explain more soon.

Thinking about thinking

Then there is thinking about thinking. This is also quite a common one but what do I mean by that? Many times, people with insomnia are at pains to point out to me that they *don't* have major problems or worries in their lives. They don't have any good reason to lie awake and it frustrates the life out of them that their mind is buzzing with all kinds of random stuff, and the thoughts keeping them awake are largely trivial. Do you do this thinking about thinking sometimes? When your mind flits around, darting from idea to idea? The trivial nature of such thoughts can become a focus in itself because it is intensely irritating to feel that you are dominated by nonsensical or unimportant thoughts. Commonly, with these types of thoughts, you may feel that you can't control your thinking, even though you are not worrying about anything in particular. Feeling that control is slipping away is not good for relaxing into sleep, but I have a good technique to share that helps block out these unimportant thoughts.

Hypervigilant thinking

This next one is about heightened awareness. We sometimes call it hypervigilance. It's as if your arousal system hasn't shut down properly and is 'looking' for things to latch on to. You could be listening in to your body and focusing on how awake you are, hearing your heartbeat thumping, or feeling an annoying itch, restlessness in your legs, or muscle tension. You get the idea – you are 'tuned into' your body, as if you are undertaking a detailed observational study of yourself. Or the hypervigilance could be toward external things like noises in the house – was that one of the children getting up? Is there someone in the house? – expansion or contraction sounds from the furniture, or it could be the wind outside, or an unfamiliar sound that you can't explain. You may even raise your head from the pillow or hold your breath to listen more intently! When your senses 'home in' on something in the still of the night it can be hard to sleep. However, this heightened awareness can be helped quite a bit by imagery training and mindfulness practices, as we shall see.

Catastrophic thoughts about sleep

This is quite a dramatic heading, isn't it? However, the mind can run away with itself in the small hours and we end up in a spiral of anxious thinking which keeps us wide awake. Catastrophic thinking about sleep, as the name suggests, is where we multiply the effects of not sleeping by focusing on the negative consequences of not sleeping. We might think,

'If I don't get to sleep soon, I will only have had a few hours' sleep', 'How am I going to get through tomorrow?', 'I'm going to make mistakes at work' and 'I'll end up being pulled up by my boss'. Imagining increasingly more catastrophic consequences of poor sleep gets us more and more upset. Our thoughts can even turn to the longer term about being stuck with insomnia, getting depressed or other unwanted health consequences. This is where rational thinking is so important. I'm going to introduce you to some techniques about thought appraisal and re-structuring to help you here.

Big picture thoughts

The final area to mention, as we come full circle in Figure 20, is what I call 'big picture' thoughts. These contrast with rehearsing and planning, which is only about the day past and the immediate next day. The big picture is about life more generally; past, present and future. A challenging situation or something important you are looking forward to may need to be thought through or resolved. There could be hurtful memories from the past or serious worries about the future. Such thoughts push to the front of our minds because they are hard to ignore. They can also feel urgent, so you stay awake trying to come up with an answer. Big picture thoughts often require some dedicated attention because there may be options to consider before you can make a decision or a plan. That's why they are really best dealt with during the day, when you were awake. Happily, there are effective strategies that can be used to solve problems and I will recommend some good ones later.

Thoughts and emotions

It is not realistic to separate our thoughts from our emotions, so I would advise you to consider how you are feeling as well as what you are thinking. That's why in the centre of Figure 20 I have emphasised both. All the different types of thoughts I have described can be associated with emotions ranging through worry, anxiety, excitement, disappointment, sadness, guilt, frustration and anger. It is this combination of thoughts and feelings that can make sleep so much more difficult. All the while of course we know that we need our sleep to help us function in life and to cope with the ups and the downs. This is one of the reasons why insomnia can be such a difficult problem to live with. You know this better than anyone! OK, so we have spent quite a bit of time on trying to understand the types of thoughts that may be causing you some trouble. What can you do to overcome your racing mind?

Putting the day to rest

As you will see in Figure 20, I think you may find this technique particularly useful for thoughts that have to do with the past day and thoughts relating to what you have on your schedule for the following day. That is, those rehearsing and planning thoughts. The aim is to put the day to bed, along with all your plans for the next day, long before bedtime . . . so that when bedtime comes you can get to sleep. If you can manage to deal with the kind of thinking that you usually do in bed before it happens, then you should sleep better.

I call this technique *putting the day to rest* or, more formally, *cognitive control*. Here is what is involved. Simply follow the steps I have summarised in Box 5. Twelve steps may seem a lot, but honestly you can do this in 10–15 minutes, no problem. You just have to make the time and get into the discipline of putting the day to rest before the evening really gets going. This may sound an easy thing to do, but because it's not something that is already part of your routine, it may be harder than you imagine. I would advise you to think through what might work for you, and then commit to a time slot that will work. Once you have put the day to rest a few times you will begin to establish this as a healthy habit, and you will likely feel the better of it as a way of separating the busy day from the evening and night to come. Remember that the thoughts that interfere at bedtime will be so much easier to dismiss if you have already dealt with them . . . and at a time when you were so much more awake to do so!

I know it may sound a bit melodramatic to talk about the racing mind as the enemy of sleep, but if we stick with the analogy of a battle for a while, then putting the day to rest is like you making the *first strike*. I mean a pre-emptive one. By getting in first, before thoughts and anxieties have the potential to bombard your night, you might be able to save yourself quite a bit of upset!

BOX 5: PUTTING THE DAY TO REST

1. Set aside 20 minutes in the early evening, the same time every night if possible (say around 7 p.m.).
2. Sit down somewhere you are not going to be disturbed.
3. All you need is something to take notes on (your laptop, a notebook), and your diary or schedule.
4. Think of what has happened during the day, how events have gone, and how you feel about the kind of day it has been.
5. Note down some of the main points. Put them to rest by committing them to print. Write down what you feel good about and also what has troubled you.
6. Write down anything you feel you need to do on a 'to do' list with steps that you can take to tie up any loose ends or unfinished business.
7. Now think about tomorrow and what's coming up. Consider things you are looking forward to as well as things that may cause you worry.
8. Write down your schedule in your diary, or check if it's already there.
9. Note down anything you are unsure about and record in your diary a time in the morning when you are going to explore that further.
10. Try to use your 20 minutes to leave you feeling more in control. Close the book on the day.

11. When it comes to bedtime, remind yourself that you have already dealt with all these things if they come into your mind.
12. If new thoughts come up in bed, note them down on a piece of paper at your bedside to be dealt with the following morning.

Giving up trying to sleep

Sometimes people are unable to sleep because they are simply overthinking sleep and trying much too hard! We spoke in Part One about *sleep attention*, *sleep intention* and *sleep effort* in this regard. Trying to fall asleep actually keeps you wakeful and leads to irritability when you don't succeed. It is understandable that you want to sleep and then try to make it happen. The drawback is that, unlike many other things in life, sleep is not something that you can *make* happen by sheer force of will. In fact, the harder you try, the less likely it is to happen. But how do you give up trying to sleep? I have found that two methods work; you can decide which of them suits you best (Table 7). You may think that I have finally taken leave of my senses! But if there is a madness in my method, there is also a method in my madness! Let me explain.

Table 7: Methods for giving up trying to sleep

Method 1 Turn the tables	Method 2 Try to stay awake
• Take every opportunity to be carefree about your insomnia.	• Lie comfortably in your bed with the lights off, but keep your eyes open.
• Relish opportunities to get out of bed whenever you can.	• Give up any effort to fall asleep.
• Try to imagine as many catastrophes as you can that will happen, just because you are awake at night. See them as exaggerated and absurd.	• Give up any concern about still being awake.
• Be prepared to accept you have insomnia. Even tell others about it.	• When your eyelids feel like they want to close, say to yourself gently 'Just stay awake for another couple of minutes, I'll fall asleep naturally when I'm ready.'
• Think of wakefulness as an opportunity, not a disaster. Use the time when you are up, to do something useful or something you enjoy.	• Don't purposefully make yourself stay awake; but if you can shift the focus off attempting to fall asleep, you will find that sleep comes naturally.

The use of *humour* is extremely powerful in helping us to take a different perspective. If we need to *de-catastrophise* a situation, that is to reduce all our exaggerated conclusions and emotions, then humour presents a good way forward. This is in part what I mean by 'turning the tables'. Try to think 'What is the worst that can happen?' and then challenge the true likelihood of all your wild imaginings. Try going with the flow instead of against it by posing less resistance to wakefulness. Accept that you will just get up if you are awake. Big deal – so do something with your extra time!

This is Method 1. It may or may not appeal to you, but I hope that you can see that a more light-hearted approach could help to reduce anxiety and effort around sleep. Patients using this approach often talk about developing a completely different attitude. Indeed, the idea of accepting situations rather than fighting them all the time has its roots in a number of ancient philosophies and religions. *Acceptance* leads to a problem having a less dominating position. Where sleep is concerned, a more mellow perspective is an adaptive outlook, and one that can lead to improved sleep.

Method 2 is an even more *paradoxical* method. In psychology we use the term *paradoxical intention* to describe therapies where you are encouraged to keep the symptom going, rather than trying to eliminate it. With insomnia you change your goal to that of staying awake, instead of getting to sleep. By deciding to stay awake you are *completely giving up trying* to sleep. When that happens, you find yourself falling asleep in spite of yourself. How reassuring it can be to find that you are overtaken by sleep! 'I don't know what happened last night, I was trying to stay awake just a few minutes longer and the next thing I knew it was morning.' That is the kind of thing that patients say when this method works for them.

The two methods have exactly the same goal – to help you give up trying to sleep. By eliminating that deliberate and focused effort, your sleep drive will strengthen and develop again naturally, and that will take you closer to your goal of being a good sleeper. I developed the sleep effort scale (SES) as a way of summarising and scoring the sleep effort problem. I have reproduced the SES for you in Figure 21.

The following seven statements relate to your night-time sleep pattern in the past week.

Please indicate by circling *one* response how true each statement is for you. Score 0 for 'not all all', 1 for 'to some extent' and 2 for 'very much', then add up your total score (maximum is 14)

1. I put too much effort into sleeping at night when it should come naturally.

   Very much   To some extent   Not at all

2. I feel I should be able to control my sleep at night.

   Very much   To some extent   Not at all

3. I put off going to bed at night for fear of not being able to sleep.

   Very much   To some extent   Not at all

4. I worry about not sleeping if I am in bed at night and cannot sleep.

Very much   To some extent   Not at all

5. I am no good at sleeping at night.

Very much   To some extent   Not at all

6. I get anxious about sleeping before I go to bed at night.

Very much   To some extent   Not at all

7. I worry about the long-term consequences of not sleeping at night.

Very much   To some extent   Not at all

Figure 21: The sleep effort scale

Why don't you fill it out just now, to represent the way you *usually* feel about your sleep? Hopefully you will see that the items in the scale reflect the habit of *sleep preoccupation* and *sleep effort* I have been talking about. Do you see from your score how much you have been overthinking your sleep? Now ask someone who is a good sleeper to fill it out. See what they score and make the comparison. I'm confident that you will find that good sleep is pretty much effort-free!

So, if overthinking sleep is part of your racing mind problem why not develop an effort-free approach by using

Methods 1 or 2 (or both)? Using our analogy of battling the enemy, this is like refusing to be provoked or bullied by sleep-related worry. That can definitely feel good!

Blocking out thoughts

I have found that people with insomnia find this technique works best with the trivial, less important thoughts that keep us awake, rather than thoughts that are to do with more worrying or more serious problems. This is the 'thinking about thinking' scenario that I described earlier and in Figure 20. If you are struggling with thoughts that flit around from topic to topic, interrupting your ability to fall over to sleep when you go to bed or when you struggle to fall back over in the middle of the night, then blocking out these thoughts could be a solution for you.

Thought-blocking involves following the three simple steps I have summarised in Box 6. I know this looks altogether too simple but using the word 'the' as a blocker is much more effective than saying to yourself to 'stop it' or telling your thoughts to 'go away'. Can't you sense the annoyance and the desperation that would be in your inner voice if you were saying 'stop' or 'go away' when under the pressure of attack from lots of unwanted pesky thoughts? This form of thought blocking is known as *articulatory suppression* and is a calm and assured way of halting the enemy advance in its tracks.

BOX 6: THREE STEPS TO SUCCESSFUL THOUGHT-BLOCKING

1. Repeat the word 'the' every 3 seconds in your head with your eyes closed.
2. Don't say it out loud, but it sometimes helps to 'mouth' it.
3. Keep up the repetitions for about 5 minutes (if you can!).

There are a couple of reasons why the method I recommend is effective. First, the word 'the' is, of course, meaningless. So, when you repeat it to yourself, over and over, it doesn't have *any* emotional effect, except maybe to bore you . . . and that might actually help! Second, thought-blocking works by stopping other thoughts from getting in. As the term suggests, it creates a block. But you might be thinking, why should doing this with the word 'the' work?

Let me give you an illustration of how a small amount of information repeated to yourself can stop other information getting to you. Suppose someone is telling you their phone number and you want to take a note of it. You don't have your phone with you to accept a shared contact, so you say thanks and go looking for a pen and paper to write the number down. Old school! All the while you are looking for the pen and pad you rehearse the number over and over to yourself. You find that mouthing (articulating) the words, but not out loud, seems to help. However, as you walk through the hallway, someone in your family is there and just says 'Hi'. What happens? You really can't respond; you can hardly even look at them . . . because 100 per cent of your mental capacity is taken up with repeating just a few numbers! The repetition blocks everything else out. It suppresses or prevents other material getting through.

This is why using something meaningless like the word 'the' can block out thoughts that might compete for your attention. Give the thought-blocking technique a good try and see how you get on with it. Thinking the word 'the' to yourself slowly and calmly every 3 seconds as you go to sleep or try to get back to sleep really helps you disconnect not only from the outside world, but importantly, also from your own thought processes.

Imagery training and mindfulness

Moving on to the next segment in Figure 20, I'm going to describe another two techniques from the 'C' part of the CBTx toolbox. I'm putting imagery training and mindfulness together here, not because they are similar to each other in what you are advised to do, but because I think they are useful for addressing the same racing mind problem, that of *hypervigilant thinking*. If your mind was a muscle, they both help you relax that muscle. When we are hypervigilant, arousal levels are high, we home in on things that feel threatening or overwhelming. In these circumstances we are prone to misperception and misinterpretation, and become overinvolved in trying to solve a problem. Typically, we end up inflating that problem all the more and just get ourselves more stressed. Imagery training and mindfulness in their different ways take you away from this frantic focus, and you land in a more peaceful place.

Let's start with *imagery training*. Imagery involves creating a mental picture, a kind of visual story in your mind. I would imagine many of you will have tried this when you can't get to sleep at night. You try thinking of something pleasant, maybe a peaceful place you know, or a holiday you enjoyed somewhere. The old idea of counting sheep and watching them jump the gate is an example of imagery. So, this is the general principle of what I mean, but there is evidence to suggest that this kind of 'thinking something up' imagery is not very effective. Maybe you have found that too? That's curious isn't it, because it sounds like distracting your frantic mind onto something that's nice should be helpful. Not so, and here's why.

I always ask people what they imagine when they try to dwell on a pleasant scene, and almost always they say that they think about being on the beach, or in a forest, or walking in the hills. Usually outdoors, usually a landscape. OK, so that's interesting, and it sounds like it could be a nice picture doesn't it? However, when I then ask them 'which beach is that?' they normally have no idea at all, or they just grab there and then for some place they know. I ask them to take me there and describe it, and at this point it becomes clear that they are struggling. They are engaged in 'thinking something up', and as I said this doesn't work.

The research data tell us that, in order to be effective, imagery should be *planned* in advance and should be well *practised*. Some of the essentials for imagery training can be found in Box 7.

BOX 7: THE ESSENTIALS OF IMAGERY TRAINING

Be prepared – don't just wait until the time comes and try to think something up. Develop a screen-play! You are the director, so shoot the scenes and edit them until you have got what you want. Your imagery sequence should take about 10 minutes to go through in your mind's eye.

Practise regularly – you are also a participant! You must learn the scenes and the sequences so that they flow as the movie rolls! You need to set time aside to learn the 'script' and you should practise in the evening or during the day too.

Get good-quality images – vivid and clear in your mind's eye is what you want. Develop the colours, the smells, the sounds, the sensations that you make part of your imagery routine.

Relax and enjoy! – who wants to watch a movie that is uninteresting? This is something that you should look forward to. But at the same time remember you want to develop an imagery story that is calming, soothing and not evocative of strong emotions!

As you can see, I want you to become the director of the movie. Develop the scenes, the settings, the participants, the sights and sounds and smells, and tell the story through the screenplay. Your goal is to create a mental film lasting about 10 minutes. Because you are the creator of it and because you are going to shoot and re-shoot it, you will get plenty of practice. By the end you will know it well, you will have learnt it, and so can easily run the reel at night. The creative piece is done and now you can settle down to enjoy and become absorbed in it. You can be on that beach, in that forest or walking in those hills. There is also the prospect of improving and adding to the imagery over time.

Now let's consider *mindfulness*. As I said this is a different approach to imagery but may also be very helpful in addressing how we approach sleep, and you may find it effective for your racing mind and your hypervigilance. Mindfulness has its origins in ancient Buddhist meditation practices but has been scientifically studied over the past 20 to 30 years, as well as becoming very popular now across the secular world. I think that mindfulness is really more of a relaxed philosophy of life with a whole system of practices, than it is a treatment. However, there are some effective mindfulness techniques that can be learnt and practised. I am going to describe a couple of exercises that I have found can be useful for insomnia.

One of these is called the 'body scan'. Don't worry it's not a medical procedure! One of the reasons I have included it is because it can easily be used when in the lying down position. That could work for sleep!

BOX 8: THE BODY SCAN

- Lie down in a comfortable position, close your eyes and draw your attention to how your body feels at this moment.

- You are supported by your bed or couch. Notice which parts of your body are in contact with the bed and which are not.

- Imagine your breathing brings energy into your body as you take some enjoyable deep breaths.

- Pay attention to your head and notice any sensations of lightness or heaviness, of warmth or coolness; whatever you experience.

- Do the same moving to your forehead . . . to your eyes . . . your nose . . . your mouth . . . your cheeks . . . your ears. Notice what you experience. Let your face soften and relax.

- Continue to sweep your attention down to your chin . . . your throat . . . your neck.
- Then to your shoulders . . . to your chest . . . each time stopping to observe, to be aware. Let every place you scan become soft.
- Become aware of your arms . . . your hands . . . your fingers lying at your side. Perhaps they are heavy, perhaps they feel light.
- Sweep now to your legs . . . to your feet . . . to your toes. Notice any pressure, notice any sensation just as it is.
- Allow your awareness to fill your whole body . . . to each part of you.
- Allow your whole body to relax and take a few more deep breaths through your nose and out through your mouth.
- Let go of any remaining tension.

As you can see in Box 8, the focus on the body is used as a way of stabilising the mind. The instructions are for you to be interested in the sensations you experience and to simply enjoy moments of sensing without thinking. The body scan is similar to the progressive relaxation and autogenic training that I describe in Chapter 11, particularly the latter, in taking your focus to various parts of your body in sequence. However, a major difference is that in the body scan there is no instruction to actively change anything. It is not about tensing or releasing muscles or about telling yourself to relax. This can be hard I know, but mindfulness is not about trying to get your hands on things to fix them. The body scan teaches you just to be mindful, to observe the sensations in a particular part of your body, to respect and accept what you experience in a manner that is kind to yourself, and at most to 'let go'. The idea is that you capture all your attention in that moment, and that is why it may be helpful in stress reduction, including during periods of hypervigilance and excessive thinking.

A second mindfulness technique that I would recommend is called the 'worry train' (Box 9). I think this approach ties in quite well with imagery because you picture yourself at a train station. Do make it a real station that you know – it makes it so much easier to imagine!

The train has lots of carriages and plenty of space for all your worries, so your task is to load the train up with the worry suitcases – the things that have been on your mind and troubling you. It's likely, as I have been saying, that your thoughts and emotions are connected, so the train has pulled in to take away your 'sad' worries as well as your 'unfair' worries, or whatever else they may be. There can be so many emotions that get attached to our thoughts, and that keep us awake! The worry train has come on schedule to take your worries away, at least for now, so that you can fall over to sleep more easily as it rolls out of the station.

As you get better at using imagery training and mindfulness practices, like the body scan and the worry train, you will find that these methods are good ways of distracting from

BOX 9: THE WORRY TRAIN

- Lie down comfortably, close your eyes and take a few deep breaths.
- Picture yourself sitting at a train station with all your luggage; each suitcase contains a different worry from your day.
- Now the train arrives; and a door opens in front of you.
- Picture yourself picking up one of the bags and taking it on to the train, loading it on the luggage rack.
- Now that your first worry is loaded – say it's worry about the future – go on to the next bag.
- Load every one of your suitcases, each with its particular worry inside.
- Finally picture yourself seated again with no luggage around you, watching the train slowly and steadily leave the station.
- You don't need to be on that train; notice how it feels to let the worry train take those worries away.

your hypervigilant self-observation, from your unwanted intrusive thoughts and emotions. These approaches capture your attention in a good way; and allow sleepiness to prevail to help you to sleep. Just like the relaxation training procedures that we cover in Chapter 11, imagery and mindfulness are not hypnotics; they don't put you to sleep, but they prepare you for sleep by putting impediments to sleep to one side. They can also be joined on to a relaxation routine, to create a longer sequence of therapeutics, and are helpful in life in general as coping and self-management skills.

Thinking rationally

When it comes to what I have called 'catastrophic thoughts', the best therapeutic approach is to use *rational thinking*. You will remember that catastrophic thinking is where your thoughts get way out of proportion, or they may not even be true at all. It is quite easy to think in a catastrophic way – especially when you are tired, sleepless, and frustrated. You might think that you are never going to get to sleep tonight or that you are going to be wrecked tomorrow; and thinking and feeling that way makes sleep harder to come and makes us feel even worse. I gave some examples a few pages ago, so it might be worth reviewing those. No doubt you will have your particular thoughts, and we will work on them shortly.

Before we do that though, let's consider rational thinking. What is that? Well, it is almost certainly what you do most of the time, because thinking rationally is considering a situation thoughtfully, analysing all the relevant information, and then arriving at a conclusion. The jargon term that we use for this process is *cognitive restructuring*. It is using your powers of reasoning, being logical, being sensible. I can almost hear you say, 'hang on, are you suggesting I'm not sensible?!' Well 'yes' and 'no' is the answer to that. I'm saying that normally you would be. That's my point. But when we get guided by our feelings and emotions, like when we are lying awake and upset, it is much harder to think that it will be fine, that you'll most likely get some sleep and that you'll manage to cope during the day. Agreed? Also, thoughts get into habits and patterns, don't they? So, after a while of repeated awakenings when you can't get back to sleep you begin to find yourself automatically thinking 'oh, no, here we go again, I'm going to struggle to sleep now'. These are negative 'automatic thoughts' and they become like a self-fulfilling prophecy.

Thinking rationally is pretty much using information to sense check what you are thinking and feeling, and it genuinely leads you to 'change your mind'. This is especially important for automatic thoughts because it's easy not to notice them. They can chip away at us if we don't deliberately spot them, and bring our reason to bear. If we learn to get into the habit of observing what we are thinking and then challenging our thoughts, beliefs and emotions, this can really help put insomnia in perspective. People who come to see me usually have been feeling out of control where sleep is concerned. They are overwhelmed by the problem, but they are also overwhelmed with their thoughts. Well,

I say to them, and now I say to you also, it is time to put you back in the driving seat. Don't be a victim of your own mind-set.

How you view your insomnia is so very important. People often tell me that insomnia has become the biggest thing in their lives. You know that I think insomnia is a 'big thing' too, otherwise I wouldn't have written this book and spent so much time researching insomnia. But . . . you absolutely *must* get out of any self-defeating perspective that leaves you feeling powerless and in its grip. You have to step firmly *towards* overcoming insomnia and move decisively *away* from a position of defeat or panic. You need to recognise that although insomnia frustrates and infuriates you, your upset and anger about it are unlikely to drive it away! Instead, we are going to see insomnia as a problem to be solved, a major problem perhaps, but nevertheless one that can be solved. Addressing the way that you are thinking is a huge step in that direction.

Have a look at Table 8. I want to help you take the fight to your insomnia by not letting it get the better of you. One effective way to do that is by thinking through your thoughts and concerns about sleep and sleeplessness *clearly* and *accurately*, and to get better at *evaluating* your thoughts. You will see that I have given you some examples of inaccurate or faulty thinking and how it might be corrected using rational thinking and cognitive restructuring. The process is:

1. to record the thought as carefully as you can
2. to consider how thinking this thought makes you feel, and to write that down

Table 8: Evaluating your thoughts and concerns about insomnia – some examples

My thoughts about sleep and sleeplessness	How this makes me feel	A more accurate version of my thoughts would be	How this version makes me feel
'It seems as if I am awake half the night and everyone else is sleeping.'	Anxious, annoyed, lonely, jealous	'I probably sleep around 6 hours and have 2 hours awake in bed; that's 75% (three-quarters) not half the night. Also if there are 1 million people living in this city and half of them are adults, maybe 50,000 are having serious problems. Everyone else is not sleeping!'	Reassured, more optimistic, less angry
'I'm never going to get to sleep tonight.'	Demoralised, out of control	'Almost certainly I will fall asleep. I always get some sleep. The average in my diary was 6 hours and I never get less than 3–4 hours.'	More accepting, relieved, more relaxed
'I'm so tired I just can't concentrate. It's because I slept so badly last night.'	Hopeless, preoccupied with sleep, irritable	'My poor concentration is not just down to my sleep. I've slept worse than I did last night and felt better during the day. Maybe I'm bored, or doing too much at once, or . . .'	More in control, able to focus

3. to re-consider the thought critically – that is, to evaluate it and to write down a new and more accurate version of the thought

4. to re-consider how thinking this new way makes you feel.

Do you get the idea? I want you to start *evaluating* your own thoughts and feelings about sleep and insomnia, as accurately as possible. I have made a blank copy of this form for you (Table 9). You should make some copies of this and keep them with your notebook; or you can find it on my www.colinespie.com website. Use this template to record the main concerns you have right now and to consider if there is another way of putting them that would be more helpful to you. Remember you can use factual information to influence what you think *and* how you feel. Follow the format I have shown you in Table 8 by putting your thoughts inside quotation marks (' . . . ') so that you realise that this is the way you are thinking. I am trying to get you to notice, record and evaluate what you are saying to yourself. It takes a bit of getting used to using this approach, but in my experience people with insomnia really benefit from first identifying their thoughts, and then evaluating them. A different mind-set really can help promote sleep.

As you do this you will realise that a lot of worry and concern over sleeplessness is based on information and beliefs that are not accurate. Negative or faulty beliefs are faulty because they are simply beliefs – that is, they are not necessarily facts. It's your responsibility to check them out

Table 9: Evaluating your thoughts and concerns about insomnia – worksheet

My thoughts about sleep and sleeplessness	How this makes me feel	A more accurate version of my thoughts would be	How this version makes me feel

– after all, they are your attributions and your beliefs – they belong to you! The good news is that faulty beliefs can be corrected, and attributions can be made more accurate. Accurate information about sleep and accurate thinking about sleep and its consequences will adjust your thoughts and feelings about your sleep . . . and will begin to modify your sleep pattern. I would go so far as to suggest that you use the thought–evaluation approach through the day so that you can write down things as they occur to you. Work away at becoming a more accurate thinker. It will be time well invested in improving your sleep, and you will feel better about yourself as well.

And speaking of time, I want to mention before moving on that *clock-watching* is not a great idea! It is often the trigger for emotional and catastrophic thinking. Have a look at Table 10. Can you see how the clock becomes a trigger that ends up with an emotional response that is arousing? Your awareness of time often gets linked to an automatic and dysfunctional thought. Because these clock thoughts also contain verbs that carry a value judgement (like 'I *should* . . . ') the next consequence is that you will evaluate yourself negatively, and this leads to a strong emotional response. Of course, an obvious solution is just to remove clocks from the bedroom! But if you do find yourself somehow monitoring time, you can use the rational thought evaluation approach (Table 9) for this too.

Table 10: The problem of clock-watching

Awareness of time	Dysfunctional thought	Self-evaluation	Emotional response
'Look at that, it's gone 12.30 . . .	*. . . and I should be well asleep by now'*	I have failed	Annoyance
'I've been lying awake for almost 2 hours now and only caught a few minutes' sleep . . .	*. . . if I don't sleep soon I'll be wrecked tomorrow'*	I have lost control	Anxiety
'Awake again . . . so what's the time now? . . . great (!) 4 a.m. . . .	*. . . I can't stand this any more; I'm going to go mad'*	I can't cope	Despair

Solving problems

The last part of Figure 20 referred to what I called 'big picture thoughts'. These are not to do with the day just past or about tomorrow, nor are they focused on how to get to sleep, or on random or relatively unimportant concerns that get out of proportion. Big picture thoughts tend to be longer lasting issues or dilemmas, and for those reasons they are not easy to dismiss or blank out. They may also be harder to think through rationally, because they may not be irrational. The problem may be a very real one and so it can command your attention in the quiet of the night. It may be that you are trying to avoid thinking about it during the daytime, or that you can't see a way through, or that you are procrastinating on something that matters. Perhaps it's too hard to contemplate so you keep busy and get on with life as best you can? However, night-time can be quite unforgiving when it comes to this type of thought. There's nothing to occupy your mind, nothing to do to keep you engaged, so the big picture thoughts come knocking at your door.

I just re-read that last paragraph, and I thought to myself that it feels rather depressing! Sorry about that. I'm trying to acknowledge that sometimes life throws hard things at us, and sleep can become a casualty – just when we need it most. The good news however is that we can do something about it, and this is where the *real-life problem-solving* approach comes in. It gives us a methodology for working our way through difficult situations, helping us to make good decisions, whilst also protecting our sleep. A bit like putting the day to rest, problem-solving is something to build into your waking life, so that bedtime hours don't become the time and place for deep thinking and action planning.

BOX 10: REAL-LIFE PROBLEM-SOLVING FOR THE 'BIG PICTURE' THOUGHTS

- Set aside 45 minutes, during the day, once per week as your real-life problem-solving time.
- Sit down somewhere private and quiet, so that you are not going to be disturbed.

- Use a notebook or device to take notes and keep track of your planned actions.

1. Consider your real-life problem. What is it exactly? Focus on one and define it carefully.

2. Consider your goal. What are you trying to achieve? Make it realistic.

3. Consider your options. What are alternative ways of achieving your goal? List at least three options.

4. Consider the 'pros' of each option. What are the positive consequences of this approach? Note them down.

5. Consider the 'cons' of each option. What are the negative consequences of this approach? Note them down.

6. Decide which option is the best one. Which alternative has the most positives and the least negative consequences? Highlight that option.

7. Decide on your action plan. What are you going to do, when, and how? Commit the plan to paper, add actions to your schedule.

8. Carry out the plan and observe the consequences. What happened and are you OK with that? Learn from your experience.

As you can see in Box 10, I recommend that you set aside time during the day for your problem-solving session. I suggest once a week should be sufficient. It is good to contain problem-solving to a planned time because then you can stop thoughts interfering at other times – you have it in hand. Also, it's best not to make decisions impulsively or when you are overly emotional so having a set time helps you to be considerate of the options and to make the best decisions on what to do next.

When we have big picture thoughts it is easy to feel overloaded mentally and overwhelmed emotionally, so I recommend that you define the problem carefully, and consider what would be a realistic goal. For example, if you have been diagnosed with a serious illness, the problem could be about acceptance of that, or consideration of treatment options that have been presented to you, or considerations about work, about finance or family factors. The problem-solving session is not about dwelling on negative events and getting upset – though you may become emotional, and that's absolutely OK and to be expected. The session is there to help you think of the problem as a challenge, to be optimistic that you are capable of developing an action plan to address the problem, and to recognise that with a bit of dedicated time and focused effort you don't need to avoid the situation. Although the life problem may be unwanted and you may wish it was not there, this approach can take you out of that sense of helplessness or hopelessness into a more positive mind-set.

I expect you will agree that it is much better to deal with

these matters in a constructive and planned way during the daytime, and if you do so, it will hugely reduce the pressure of such big picture thoughts on your racing mind at night.

Well, that takes us through the reasons why our minds might not turn off at night and my suggested solutions for each type of troublesome thought. I hope that one or more of these techniques works for you. Make sure to give them a good try out! Thinking habits in bed are just like any other kind of habit, and you may have got into the way of thinking, thinking, thinking when your head hits the pillow. You have to stem the flow of the thoughts from being there in the first place, manage them differently when they do occur, and break those old thought habits. Then I'm confident you will be on the way to being a good sleeper again!

Establishing Your New Sleep Pattern – Behavioural Therapeutics

Introduction

Here we find ourselves at the 'B' in CBT, the behavioural part. Whether you came straight here from Table 6 and the associated text, or came in after working on your racing mind or your arousal, you are most welcome! In this chapter, we will be looking at your sleep pattern and how to get it into the best possible shape, and how to keep it that way. I'm sure this chapter is going to be relevant for you, but it will be particularly suited if you need a re-build of your sleep pattern. There are two main ways to achieve that rebuild and you have the choice of how to go about it.

The chapter is divided into two main sections (Figure 22). The first section focuses on strengthening the connection between bed and successful sleep. This will be particularly helpful if you find that going to bed seems to

Strengthening your bed-sleep connection	Improving your sleep efficiency
For many people with insomnia being in bed is associated with lying awake, stressed, tossing and turning. The bed should be a place of rest, relaxation and sleep.	Many people with insomnia have a low sleep efficiency. Across the night, hours and hours are spent lying awake, such that the proportion of the night spent asleep is too low.
This section helps you re-establish the connection that the good sleeper has between bed and getting to sleep quickly.	This section helps you to develop a high sleep efficiency so that your sleep pattern can knit back together again.

Figure 22: Behavioural therapeutics

wake you up, and that lying awake is a stressful experience. I will teach you techniques that help to re-establish a strong bond between being in bed and getting to sleep quickly. In the second section, I focus on helping you to improve your 'sleep efficiency'. You will remember that sleep efficiency is the amount of sleep that you get, divided by the time you spend in bed, expressed as a percentage. So, 6 hours sleep and 8 hours in bed is three-quarters or 75 per cent. If your sleep efficiency is below 80 per cent, you have a lot of wake time in bed, so I will explain ways that you squeeze that wakefulness out of the night!

Establishing your new sleep pattern is about improving your bed–sleep connection and getting your sleep efficiency higher so you can sleep through the night. You can start with either approach, and they also work well together, so it's up to you. In the insomnia world, therapy for the bed–sleep connection is known as *stimulus control* and therapy for sleep efficiency is known as *sleep compression* or *sleep restriction* therapy. I will explain these rather complex terms in simple language, so that you are clear about what you are meant to do. I believe that these approaches are particularly powerful components of CBT, so I'm optimistic that we can make good progress.

The purpose of these behavioural therapeutics then is to *reshape your sleep so that it meets your individual needs and develops into a strong pattern that will last*. Looking forward to getting going!

Strengthening the connection between bed and sleep

I like to use the word *connection* when I explain stimulus control to my patients. You don't need to understand the origins or the details of this technical term, you just need to know that it is about connection. So, what do I mean by connection? Try to picture this in your mind. I'm imagining a firm bond that is guaranteed by a powerful adhesive, or I'm thinking of a strong chain where the links are solidly connected even when the chain is under strain. The type of connection I am recommending then is one that you can rely on. It's not a loose connection like you might get with faulty wiring, or a remote connection where you perhaps know someone only through a mutual acquaintance. The kind of connection I am referring to is a union that is hard to break.

This is the starting point for your new sleep pattern. It's about strengthening the connection between bed and sleep. So, let's turn to that. Let's consider what is the connection between bed and sleep for you? Could it do with being strengthened? These are probably hard questions, and you are probably wondering what I am talking about! Let's start with an easier question. What do you think is the connection between bed and sleep for the good sleeper? They go to bed and they sleep through the night. The good sleeper thinks of 'bed' and immediately thinks 'sleep'. Bed means sleep. You go to bed – you fall asleep. Bed is a place for . . . sleeping. Can you see what I mean? Bed to the good sleeper is strongly connected to sleep.

So back to you. What is the connection between bed and sleep in your experience? Well, I suppose it could be a number of things, but I could hazard a few guesses. You think of 'bed' and you think 'groan' or think and worry 'what if I don't sleep'. You might even have a kind of phobia about going to bed. Bed means for you lying awake tossing and turning. Thinking about going to bed makes you anxious. Bed means . . . a long shift till morning comes. You go to bed – you lie awake, you try to fill in the time somehow. Bed is a place . . . for sleeping, yes at times . . . but often you don't sleep, so the connection with sleep is weak.

I'm thinking that your bed–sleep connection may be broken. Indeed, you likely have a bed–wake connection at the moment because being in bed is associated time and time again with difficulty getting to sleep or getting back to sleep. This is what we call *conditioning*. Things get paired together. Your bed is connected with your insomnia not with sleep, and this is why we need to reconnect your bed with successful sleep. We need to re-establish that connection. This is *re-conditioning*. We want to get you back to being a good sleeper whose sleep comes quickly in bed. It will be so much easier for you to get to sleep and to remain asleep if your mind and your body automatically make a *sleep response* to an important *cue*: your bed. That is how it is for the good sleeper – cue bed, cue sleep! That is where you want to be, I'm sure.

There are a number of things I can suggest that will help create a strong connection between your sleep and your bed.

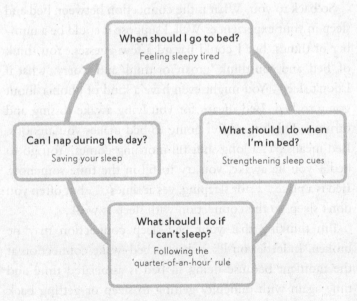

Figure 23: Establishing a strong bed–sleep connection

In Figure 23 I have addressed four common questions, each of which relates to the bed–sleep connection. You will see that against each question I have suggested a behavioural therapeutic that will help reconnect and strengthen that connection. I think all four will be useful to you, but you might want to read through the questions and the treatment techniques so you can decide where to start your behavioural treatment.

Feeling sleepy tired

This is the answer to the question *'When should I go to bed?'* It is important that you only go to bed when you feel sleepy enough to get to sleep quickly. If you are not sleepy when you go to bed it is quite unlikely that you will fall asleep. Don't you think? This is especially true if you have been finding that you become even more awake as soon as you get into bed. You need to be sleepy enough for the build-up of your sleep drive to carry you into your sleep. The same thing applies during the night if you waken up and can't get back to sleep. You will see a little further down that I recommend you get up if you are unsuccessful in returning to sleep. At those times too, I advise you to return to bed when you feel sleepy enough to sleep.

I wonder if you remember as a child saying to your parents ' . . . *but I'm not tired!'* You wanted to stay up later than usual to watch the TV, but your mum or dad said that it was 'past your bedtime'. Is this ringing a bell? You would try to look wide awake, and definitely try to resist any sign that you were sleepy! Or you might complain once you were in your bed *'I can't get to sleep!'* because, although you were in bed, you were not sleepy enough to fall over? OK, sometimes going to bed, or being 'sent' to bed could be a bit of a battleground, couldn't it? Maybe these days the battle repeats itself with you and your own children, or grandchildren even! However, I hope you are understanding my simple point, that it is hard to sleep if you are not sleepy.

All that happens if you find yourself lying awake in your bed, is that you break that connection between bed and sleep, and you build up a lot of frustration in the process. If you want to repair the bed–sleep connection, make sure you are sleepy when you decide to go to bed. I want to help you to see that this involves two important things. First, you need to recognise poor reasons for deciding to go to bed; and second, you need to be able to recognise what sleepiness actually is!

BOX 11: GO TO BED WHEN YOU FEEL 'SLEEPY TIRED', NOT FOR OTHER REASONS

Poor reasons for deciding to go to bed (when you have insomnia)	Feeling 'sleepy tired': the best reasons for deciding to go to bed
It's late, it's past my bedtime	I'm struggling to stay awake
I've finished watching the TV	I'm yawning

There's nothing else to do	I've already nodded off
My partner is going to bed	I've lost track of what I was doing
I need to get up early tomorrow	Other people have noticed that I'm sleepy
I need to catch up on lost sleep	My eyes are itchy and I'm rubbing them
I slept really badly last night	My muscles ache and I need to stretch

Once you get your sleep back into a good routine and you are sleeping well you won't need to think about this too much. However, for now, consider the possibility that you are going to bed for the 'wrong' reasons and most importantly that you are failing to take your cue for bed-time from your own sleepiness. In Box 11 I have given you seven examples of poor reasons for going to bed, and seven examples of the best reasons for going to bed. The main difference between the sets of examples (and they are just examples) is that if your *sleepiness decides* when it's time to go to bed you will likely fall asleep; whereas if *you decide* there is no good reason why you should fall asleep at that time of your choice. I appreciate that you may like to go to bed at a regular time, or when your partner goes to bed, and you may not wish to stay up with nothing much to do, but as I say that's for the future. Right now, I want you to get the act of going to bed firmly associated with successful and rapid sleep-onset.

I have used the term *sleepy tired*. Let me just clarify this, because you need to be able to differentiate symptoms and signs of being sleepy (e.g. yawning and a tendency to 'nod off') and feelings of tiredness when it occurs on its own. Tiredness does not mean that sleep is inevitable, whereas sleepiness is a signal from our bodies that it is time for our night's sleep. We might be lacking in energy or feeling fatigued but still not be ready to sleep, so work on this a bit and see if you can identify clear signs of sleepiness that are typical for you. Be reassured that once you are a good sleeper again, going to bed will be able to trigger sleepiness. We need to rebuild the bed–sleep connection that at the moment is broken.

Strengthening sleep cues

Sleepiness as we have seen is the most important sleep cue, but people often ask *'what should I do when I'm in bed'?* They are interested in understanding bedtime activities that are 'allowed' and that are likely to help them sleep, differentiating them from activities that are likely to keep them awake. This is the next component of our programme for strengthening the bed–sleep connection.

People get quite obsessed with this one in my experience. Indeed, if you don't have clarity on what to do and what not to do in bed you may become anxious. Perhaps that's because our bedtime routine has a long personal history. When you were a child you may have had your 'comforter' that you took to bed with you. It was the thing that enabled you to form a *comfort bridge* between wakefulness, being in bed, and sleep. The soft toy, piece of fabric, soother/pacifier, or thumb helped you to settle in bed. Its physical presence, even its smell, allowed you to close your eyes. Without it you might not have been able to sleep, and you might have become distressed. Perhaps it was an object that was reserved for bedtime or sleep time? Although your parents never used the theoretical framework, they had discovered this object was a powerful stimulus or trigger to the conditioning of your bedtime behaviour and to your automatic settling to sleep response.

I hear you say, but that's for children; I'm not a child anymore. Too true. However, you are still conditioned. We all are. That is why the bed–sleep connection works for the good sleeper. Head hits pillow – cue sleep – and sleep responds. So often people with insomnia point out the opposite, that when their head hits the pillow – zing, they are wide awake. They observe that their partner 'goes out like a light', but they do not. I rest my case on the principle, we are all conditionable.

The pillow example is a great one because here we have the same thing – a pillow – for one person triggering sleep, yet for another person triggering wakefulness. From this it becomes clear that it is not the object or the activity itself that is important, but whether it acts to strengthen or weaken the individual's relationship with sleep.

Let me take another example, that of reading in bed. Most treatment manuals say that people with insomnia should not read in bed, because reading is a waking activity and that reading keeps you awake. The suggestion is that reading is incompatible with sleep, and that reading should take place in a waking environment, like the living-room, and should be banned from the bedroom and being in bed. You can see that this makes sense. Reading should be associated with a place where we are awake because we need to be awake to read. However, many of my patients have heard this and, quite rightly, say 'but my partner reads in bed and it doesn't interfere with sleep. My partner doesn't have insomnia; why can't I read in bed?' As with the pillow, it is the association that matters. For many good sleepers reading is not associated with insomnia. The good sleeper reads in bed with the intention of reading – that is, their intention is to remain awake in order to read. So, reading in bed is associated if anything with an effort to remain awake. Contrast that with the poor sleeper, who is actually using reading as a tool to get to sleep and *doesn't* wish to be awake. Good sleepers struggle to remain awake to read and so reading becomes associated with sleep being powerful. Poor sleepers just find that reading becomes associated with more frustration and stress!

My point is this, there are general 'rules' for what to do and what not to do when you are in bed, but they need to be personally tailored so that they strengthen your behaviour in bed as a cue for sleep rather than as a cue for continued wakefulness. To overcome your insomnia, it is very important that in rebuilding your sleep pattern you get into the way of *falling asleep very rapidly* after you get into bed. I want you to develop a quick bed/sleep response. I have explained this in Table 11.

Table 11: Strengthening cues to sleep when you are in bed

	Bedtime behaviour	What the behaviour cues or signals
Strengthening	Putting out the light	End of the waking day
	Adopting your sleeping position	Transition from waking to sleep
	Closing your eyes	Intention to sleep
	Relaxing	Letting go
	Chatting with your partner	Neutral, but likely pro-sleep
	Sexual activity	
Weakening	Reading	Continued waking activity / Social engagement / Work mode / Emotional activation
	Watching TV	
	Speaking on the phone	
	Engaging in social media	
	Catching up on emails	
	Gaming	

I strongly recommend that when you go to your bed, you should put the light out straight away and put your head down intending to sleep. This is a good time to relax and 'let go' to release yourself into sleep. If you are also following my recommendation about going to bed when you are sleepy tired, there is no good reason to continue activities that, at least until you have overcome your insomnia, are likely to weaken the bed–sleep connection. Besides, as you can see in Table 11, many of these behaviours serve as signals not just to remaining awake, but also to increased arousal and emotion. I regard chatting with your partner and sexual activity as exceptions to this rule. They are more likely sleep enablers because they bring closure and comfort to the day and usually help us sleep.

What should I do if I can't sleep?

You might be thinking all this is well and good but what if I go to bed sleepy, try to get to sleep but can't? What do I do then?

This is where what I call the *quarter of an hour rule* comes in. I completely understand, and expect, that there will be nights when you put your head down and sleep will not come quickly. What I recommend here is that if sleep does not come within quarter of an hour, you should get out of bed and go into another room. Think again of the importance of the bed–sleep connection. By getting up from bed you keep wakeful time associated with a wakeful environment in the house. Importantly, you also get out of that habit of lying in bed and getting frustrated. If you are not sleeping, you are not sleeping. It is as simple as that. Stop trying to sleep. That will simply get you more wound up. Get up and break that cycle because sleep will come when it is ready, and then you can go back to bed when you are sleepy again. I have summarised how to put the quarter of an hour rule into practice in Box 12.

BOX 12: WHAT TO DO IF YOU CAN'T SLEEP: PUTTING THE QUARTER OF AN HOUR RULE IN PRACTICE

Instructions for the quarter of an hour rule

1. Trust that you can estimate quarter of an hour approximately.

2. Don't use a clock, watch or device to monitor time.
3. Give yourself the opportunity to sleep, or to get back to sleep if its during the night.
4. If you think quarter of an hour has passed get up and execute your waking plan.
5. When you feel sleepy again go back to bed.
6. Trust once again that you can estimate quarter of an hour approximately.
7. Repeat steps 1–6 as often as necessary across the night.

Before you go to bed set up your waking plan

- Have somewhere to go
- Have something to do
- Have something to keep you warm and comfortable
- Have something to drink at hand

I know that, just like being awake when it seems like everyone else is sleeping, getting out of bed when you want to sleep is going to be very difficult! It may be hard because you feel cosy and don't want to leave the warmth of the bed. It may be hard because you worry you will wake everyone else up. It may be hard to know what to get up and do. But there are things that will make getting out of bed easier

– you could leave the heating on and a table lamp on in your living room. You could prepare a warm milky drink or a decaffeinated drink and put it in a flask at your armchair before you go to bed – because you know you *will* be awake tonight. You could read or listen to music or do something else that is relaxing while you are up. People often ask me if it needs to be a boring book. To which I reply that I wonder why on earth anyone would want to read a boring book?! No, the idea is that you are content to get up and can enjoy doing something else for a while. You can also discuss your plan with your partner and get support and agreement that the plan is OK to implement. If you absolutely can't get up from bed, or don't have another room to go to, I recommend that you sit upright in bed and follow your plan to occupy yourself for a while *until you feel sleepy again* and want to lie back down.

Think of it like this, the more that you get up when you are not sleeping, and the more you return to bed when you feel sleepy again, the more likely it is that you will fall asleep quickly on returning to bed. This applies both when you can't get to sleep at first, and if you can't get back to sleep during the night. If you still cannot sleep when you go back to bed, you will need to get out of bed yet again! So, let's imagine that you put the quarter of an hour rule into practice two or three times a night for one week, that could be fifteen to twenty times you have broken the bed–wake connection and re-established the bed–sleep connection. It can begin to work quickly. It's like re-booting the system towards quickly and successfully getting to sleep.

Before moving on to the next section, let me explain a little bit more about why I am emphasising this idea of quarter of an hour. First, there's very strong evidence that good sleepers fall asleep within 15 minutes or so. Therefore, if you want to become a good sleeper, you need to train yourself to fall asleep within a short timeline. Quarter of an hour is long enough to fall asleep at the beginning of the night or during the night. Second, and following from this, if you extend that *sleep opportunity* into a half-hour or longer you will have less and less success. Third, I use the term quarter of an hour because I want to emphasise giving yourself a short opportunity. I definitely don't mean 15 minutes! I absolutely don't want you to count down the clock. Besides, you can tell the time without a watch or a clock. If my dog can tell the time, then I'm sure you can! Without fail, he knows when it's dinner time and goes and sits by his bowl, just like clockwork. Trust yourself to know when you have given sleep a chance. Finally, you don't need to wait as long as that if you don't want to. If you don't feel sleepy it's OK to get up sooner. This quarter of an hour rule is simply an *estimate* of the time after which you should be getting up. Remember, if it's good enough for good sleepers, it's good enough for you too.

Can I nap during the day?

The final thing to do to strengthen the connection between night-time sleep and your bed is to avoid napping during the day – or in the evening. I want to emphasise the importance of remembering that bed is for sleep and night is for sleep. *Daytime is for wakefulness.* This is a fundamental principle. If your sleep seeps into the daytime it is likely that being awake will seep into your night, and this will only make your insomnia worse. Stopping naps if you are in the habit of taking them will not only better prepare you for a continuous, longer sleep at night but will strengthen the connection between your bed and sleep. Sleeping in a chair in another room weakens that important link.

BOX 13: NAPPING AND SAVING YOUR SLEEP FOR NIGHT-TIME

- Save your sleep for the night-time.
- Avoid naps during the day or evening if at all possible.
- Keeping active can help resist the tendency to feel tired and sleepy.
- Recognise that tiredness/fatigue and sleepiness are different things.
- If you do need to sleep, keep the nap brief (10 minutes).
- Consider whether your lifestyle is resulting in you being sleep deprived.
- If you struggle to remain awake during the day or fall asleep without intending to, seek advice.

In Figure 23, I referred to this as *saving your sleep* and in Box 13 I have summarised my advice about naps. It's a bit like saving yourself to enjoy your meals by not snacking in between. The way the sleep-wake schedule is organised we are designed to sleep at night and to be awake during the day, so the more that we can live by that rule of biology the better we will feel. At times this involves resisting the temptation to sleep, just like resisting the temptation to snack! If we think about it in a developmental context, babies and toddlers have daytime sleeps and that is normal for their age and stage of development. However, by the time a 5-year-old is at school, napping during the day has disappeared and is not provided for in the curriculum in the way that it would have been at nursery or kindergarten. Likewise, in adult life, napping during the day is not necessary, although in some cultures and climates people do have a break in activities. The siesta is a short nap that is traditionally taken in the early afternoon after a meal.

You might be thinking then, why should I not have a nap if it doesn't cause insomnia in those situations? In response to that common question, I would point out that in Mediterranean regions people traditionally go to bed considerably later, and this may be partly due to the fact that their sleep drive is delayed by the nap. They also have their main meal later in the evening, so their lifestyle patterns are adjusted across the day and evening times. We also know that the effect of a nap on your night-time sleep will be affected by nap duration. Typically, a short nap of say 10 minutes will have less impact on your ability to fall asleep at night than a longer nap. Longer naps of course can turn into daytime sleeps, and if you get into deep sleep during the day you will find it's a struggle to waken again and it will feel less restorative when you waken because you will experience some *sleep inertia*. This is a feeling of grogginess that continues until you have properly woken up.

So, whether you nap or not is up to you. Generally, I advise against it when you are trying to overcome your insomnia, because it makes sense to save your sleep for night-time. You can try to keep yourself active during the day; and take some planned exercise if you feel tired. However, there are some circumstances in which I do think it is important to consider taking a nap.

If you feel that you absolutely must have a nap, or if you regularly fall asleep without wanting to, then it is important to consider why that might be. Possibilities include being sleep deprived by not having the opportunity to get enough sleep, say through pressure of work or jet lag; and having another type of sleep problem that is more associated with excessive daytime sleepiness than insomnia is. I covered this in some detail in the assessment chapter (Chapter 6) and there is more information to come in Part Four. You should also consider your safety and that of others if you are struggling to remain awake when you are driving. Trying to resist symptoms of sleepiness is not very effective. You should pull over, have some strong coffee and take a nap before continuing. The coffee takes a little while to 'hit' as a stimulant. So, in those circumstances a 10-minute nap first helps restore your alertness and the coffee effect kicks in after you waken up.

Table 12: Making decisions about the bed–sleep connection

Decisions I have made about bedtime activities	Decisions I have made about the quarter-of-an-hour rule	Decisions I have made about feeling sleepy	Decisions I have made about avoiding napping

If you continue to feel sleepy enough to fall asleep without wanting to during the day, or it is affecting your ability to remain awake, you should think through why you are so sleepy and get professional advice and assessment if required. Naps are only ever a very temporary fix, so don't become dependent on them.

Summary of the bed–sleep connection

I know that I have been hitting you hard with a lot of rules right now, so let's just take stock for a moment. This is all about strengthening the bed–sleep connection so that it becomes reliable and automatic, like it is for the good sleeper. That won't be easy, and I need your commitment to help make it happen. This is why, in Table 12, I have left space for you to write down any decisions that you face concerning each element of the bed–sleep connection. Take some time to think through how you are going to apply each of these rules. Try not to kid yourself that you will 'just do it' – you won't! This part of the CBT programme is very challenging, so you need to consider carefully how you are going to achieve success in putting this aspect of your new sleep pattern into practice.

Improving your sleep efficiency

This section on behavioural therapeutics focuses on improving your sleep efficiency. We need to work out how much sleep you need and how you can manage to get that same amount of sleep on a night-to-night basis. More than that we want your sleep to be good quality sleep, and for most people that means falling asleep quickly and sleeping through the night. But let's take a closer look at what sleep efficiency is and how it can be addressed using this part of the 'B' in CBT. I introduced you to this term in Part One; and said a bit more about it when we spoke about 'Your Data' as part of the RAPIDLY framework. Sleep efficiency is a data point; it's a useful measure, so let's make sure we understand what it means and then I'll show you a few ways that you can calculate your own sleep efficiency.

What is sleep efficiency?

People with insomnia are inefficient sleepers. That is, they only sleep for part of the night, whereas good sleepers sleep for most of it. Look at the examples in Box 14.

BOX 14: NAPPING AND SAVING YOUR SLEEP FOR NIGHT-TIME

Mia goes to bed at 11 p.m. and gets up at 7 a.m. She sleeps all of the 8 hours between these times. This means that Mia is a very efficient sleeper indeed – in fact she has **100 per cent** *sleep efficiency* because she sleeps absolutely all of the time she spends in bed.

Callum also goes to bed at 11 p.m. and gets up at 7 a.m. He takes 45 minutes to fall asleep and is awake

---

during the night for another 90 minutes. This means that Callum is awake for 2 hours 15 minutes. He sleeps for 5 hours 45 minutes of the 8 hours that he is in bed. Callum's sleep efficiency therefore is only **72 per cent**.

What do you think about Mia? She looks like she is a perfect sleeper. If you were like her, falling asleep immediately and never waking up at all till morning, then getting out of bed as soon as you woke up, your sleep efficiency would be 100 per cent. That's not going to happen, even for the good sleeper, so Mia really doesn't exist! However, most good sleepers can manage around 90 per cent sleep efficiency; that is, about 10 per cent of their time in bed is spent awake. Let's do the arithmetic here. This would be the equivalent of spending 8 hours in bed (480 minutes), and only having a total of 48 minutes (10 per cent) throughout that whole time awake. That sounds more achievable doesn't it? Even good sleepers take a little while to get sleep, have some wakeful minutes through the night, and also lie in bed for a while in the morning before they get up.

Now let's look at Callum's experience. He is in bed for the same amount of time as Mia, but Callum has difficulty getting to sleep and staying asleep. It all adds up to 135 minutes, and this results in his sleep efficiency being rather low at 72 per cent. I imagine this looks and feels more like your sleep pattern right now? Fragmented sleep like this is a terrible experience; and it doesn't set you up well for the day!

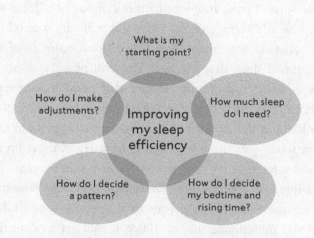

Figure 24: Improving your sleep efficiency

Have a look now at Figure 24. Here I have laid out your programme for improving your sleep efficiency. First, we will address your starting point, by finding out what your sleep efficiency is right now. Then we will move on to thinking about how much sleep you are getting and how much you need. After that we will think about your night-time schedule, before moving on to consider how we get your sleep into an efficient and effective pattern. Finally, we will think about adjustments you can make along the way to keep things going in the right direction.

Working out your own sleep efficiency

The first method of calculating your sleep efficiency is a quick, ready reckoner, if you like. It's one that you can do right now. Take a moment to think about how long you sleep on the average night. I know it will vary a good bit, but what do you think would be a good estimate of the amount of sleep that you get? You will probably think of this in hours and minutes so take that number, convert it into minutes, and put that in the left box in Figure 25. Now think about the amount of time you usually spend in bed, from when you climb into bed until when you get up the final time. Again, it's an estimate and it's an average. Put that figure in minutes into the middle box. You now have an equation. By dividing your total sleep by your time in bed and multiplying that by 100 you well get a calculation of your sleep efficiency. Write that figure into the sleep efficiency % box on the right.

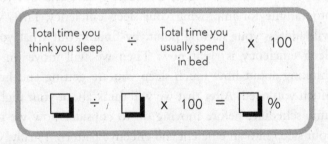

Figure 25: Estimating your sleep efficiency using a calculator

I'm sure you will have an immediate reaction to the figure. If it's higher than you thought, all to the good. If it's lower, well just remember why you are here. That's the problem we are trying to solve!

I have provided you with another sense check on your sleep efficiency in Figure 26. Here you can 'look up' your sleep efficiency by reading across (how much sleep are you getting) and reading down (how long are you spending in bed). This will take you to a value that is your estimated sleep efficiency. Circle the value you get to and compare it with what you had from your previous calculation. I expect they are the same or similar. You should also be able to see, from Figure 26, how far below 90 per cent your sleep efficiency is, and also what kind of 'banding' of sleep quality it relates to.

You will be able to use the sleep efficiency value that you have now as your baseline. This is your starting point if you like and we will be working towards improving it towards that 90 per cent mark. However, if you have been completing the sleep diary that I recommended in Part Two, you can get a more precise measurement of sleep efficiency from your diary data. We will come to that shortly.

How much sleep do I need?

How much sleep do you *need*? The amount of sleep that you need may well be different from the amount of sleep that you want. It is likely also to be different from what the average amount of sleep is for a man or woman of your age. We spoke about this in Part One, and recognised that everyone's sleep needs differ, so there is not a single answer to

Hours	3	3.5	4	4.5	5	5.5	6	6.5	7	7.5	8	8.5	9	9.5	10
3	100														
3.5	86	100													
4	75	88	100												
4.5	67	78	89	100											
5	60	70	80	90	100										
5.5	55	64	73	82	91	100									
6	50	58	67	75	83	92	100								
6.5	46	54	62	69	77	85	92	100							
7	43	50	57	64	71	79	86	93	100						
7.5	40	47	53	60	67	73	80	87	93	100					
8	37	44	50	56	63	69	75	81	88	94	100				
8.5	35	41	47	53	59	65	71	76	82	88	94	100			
9	33	39	44	50	56	61	67	72	78	83	89	94	100		
9.5	32	37	42	47	53	58	63	68	74	79	84	89	95	100	
10	30	35	40	45	50	55	60	65	70	75	80	85	90	95	100

Total sleep time (hours)

Sleep efficiency %

Time in bed (hours)

Figure 26: Estimating sleep efficiency chart

the question. For example, you might have a shorter sleep requirement than some other people. Although you might prefer to have brown eyes instead of blue, or to be taller or shorter in height, you will know that these are things you can't change. There's nothing 'wrong' with them. They are just individual differences. What is more, your sleep needs will have changed over the course of your lifetime. Unfortunately, my dark brown hair has long since been grey! You have to be prepared to adjust your expectations about sleep, and so your sleep behaviour, accordingly. All this said, however, I am very confident that your sleep pattern will work best for you when you accept you have to work within whatever natural boundaries are there for you now. So, we are going to spend a bit of time discovering what your personal sleep needs are.

Insomnia poses a particular challenge in working out how much sleep you need. This is because at the moment your sleep is likely to be upset in a way that makes each night different. For example, a person with insomnia may sleep 4 or 5 hours some nights, while on other nights manage to get 6 or 7 hours. In one way or another, insomnia is often a mix of bad nights and better nights, which is pretty frustrating! Another common problem is that difficulties getting to sleep and waking in the night break the sleep that you do get into bits. This will make it feel like you have had even less sleep, even if the total time, added up, doesn't look so bad.

BOX 15: CALCULATING YOUR AVERAGE SLEEP TIME

Night	Amount of time I slept
1	
2	
3	
4	
5	
6	
7	
8	
9	
10	

Total amount of sleep over 10 days ....

My average sleep time ....

I imagine that it may be hard for you to know how much sleep you need, especially if your pattern is all over the place. Here's what I suggest in my clinic as the best way to find out how much sleep you need: using your sleep diary it is quite easy to work out how much sleep you are getting, on average. First, write down in the spaces in Box 15 the amount of time you think you actually slept in total for each of the last ten nights. Second, add up the total time you have slept across these nights and write that in. Third, divide the total by ten to note down the *average length of your night's sleep*.

Before we move on to the next step, it is worth saying that you will probably have come up with a figure that is considerably less than what you are aiming at. But this is just your starting point. So far, we have only found out how much sleep you are getting. Remember that no matter how little sleep that adds up to, it will still be worthwhile sleep.

Follow the programme with me and you will see how you can first of all get rid of your difficulties getting to sleep and staying asleep, and after that you can build up your total sleep time to the amount of sleep you actually need.

Deciding your bedtime and rising time

Your next goal is to work out a way of achieving the *same* amount of sleep *every* night. This is important because we should be aiming for a sleep pattern that you can rely upon – that is, one that is stable and does not vary much from night to night. We know that good sleepers can rely on having a consistent pattern, so this should be your goal, too.

We have found out the average amount of sleep that you have been getting. Now I want you to get this same amount every night, but in one continuous sleep. In other words, to get you sleeping right through!

Deciding on Your Rising Time

Now let's decide on a rising time or getting-up time. It is best to have a set time for getting up every morning, seven nights a week, until you get your sleep problem sorted. I always recommend that you should *anchor* your sleep around this *fixed morning rising time*. This anchoring is to stop your sleep from drifting and to help it to settle down to a reliable pattern. To do this, you should now choose a time in the morning that you will rise from bed. The time you choose is up to you, but it should be a time that you are comfortable with and that allows you to do all the things you need to do during the day. For example, you may find that 6:30 or 7:00 a.m. is good because during the week you need to get up at that time for work.

You should now have both your average sleep time and your fixed morning rising time, but before we firm up on the rising time, there's one more thing to consider – bedtime. At the moment, how do you decide when to go to bed?

Deciding on Your Bedtime

Sometimes people go to bed before they are sleepy tired and end up lying awake, or they fall asleep quickly but wake up too early. At other times, people will go to bed early to try to catch up on the sleep they have lost on previous nights. As we were saying in the section on feeling 'sleepy tired' (and Box 11) people sometimes go to bed because 'everyone else has gone to bed', or just because 'it's bedtime'. People even force themselves to stay up very late or do strenuous workouts in an effort to exhaust themselves, in the belief that this will make them sleep better.

However, the answer to the question 'When should I go to bed?' is fairly straightforward. You should go to bed at a time which makes it likely that you will sleep right through the night. The next step, then, is to set what I call a *threshold time* for going to bed. This is to mark the point at which you are able to cross the threshold from waking to sleeping. It is worked out by subtracting your average sleep time from your morning rising time.

Let's take an example to show how this works. If Charlie had estimated that he was sleeping 5½ hours and had planned for a fixed rising time of 7 a.m., then his threshold time to go to bed would be 1.30 a.m. (7 a.m less 5½ hours). However, some flexibility can be useful, because he might prefer to get up a bit earlier so as not to be so late to bed. Charlie then might instead set a rising time of 6.00 a.m., and the threshold time would then be adjusted to 12.30 a.m. I hope this makes sense. As long as you set a tight 'sleep window' based on your total sleep then you can make that decision about establishing the fixed rising time and the threshold time.

Threshold time

Fixed rising time	10:30	11:00	11:30	12:00	12.30	01:00	01:30	02:00	02.30	03:00
08.30	10	9.5	9	8.5	8	7.5	7	6.5	6	5.5
08:00	9.5	9	8.5	8	7.5	7	6.5	6	5.5	5
07.30	9	8.5	8	7.5	7	6.5	6	5.5	5	
07:00	8.5	8	7.5	7	6.5	6	5.5	5		
06:30	8	7.5	7	6.5	6	5.5	5			
06:00	7.5	7	6.5	6	5.5	5				
05:30	7	6.5	6	5.5	5					
05:00	6.5	6	5.5	5						

Fixed rising time

Figure 27: Selecting your best sleep window

With all this in mind then, and using your own data, have a look at the chart in Figure 27. On the diagonal lines you will see your sleep window options. These range from 5 hours through to 10 hours. I expect the amount of sleep that you estimate you are getting right now will be at the lower end of that range! If you look up and down the diagonal you will be able to read off the choices that you have about your fixed rising time and your threshold time. You are free to select whatever option suits you best. Once you have decided your sleep window, write the rising time and threshold time down in Box 16.

BOX 16: YOUR FIXED RISING TIME
AND YOUR THRESHOLD TIME FOR
CONSIDERING GOING TO BED

My preferred sleep window:

Fixed rising time: _____

Threshold time: _____

Please remember that your threshold time is *not* your actual bedtime. Your time for going to bed must always be at, or after, the threshold. Your threshold time is the *earliest* you can go to bed. I want you to monitor how sleepy tired you feel and then to go to bed when you feel sleepy tired. That needs to be after you get to the threshold.

How do I establish a pattern?

You may be thinking, 'Surely, he doesn't mean that I have to do this every night, including weekends?' Sorry, the answer is yes, I'm asking you to make this a nightly schedule, at least for now. If you have been struggling with your sleep pattern over past months, and perhaps even years, then taking a seven-nights-a-week approach to sorting it is going to be necessary. Your threshold time and your rising time are meant for every day of the week, and this is why this technique is commonly called sleep restriction. It is challenging, but it really does work.

Imagine if you slept right through from the moment your head hit the pillow until the moment your alarm clock went off – you would be sleeping 100 per cent of the night! The programme I have described for you actually gives you the chance of reaching that 100 per cent, at least some nights, because the homeostatic pressure for sleep (your sleep drive) will build up as you follow the programme every night. Sleep inevitably will fill in the only gap you make available to it – your new sleep window. In practice, though, I want to help you to increase your sleep efficiency to around 90 per cent, and certainly into the 80–90 per cent range if it was very low to start with. That is an achievable goal. I accept that weekends will be hard for you, so use your alarm clock to make sure you rise at your fixed time.

How do I make adjustments?

I want to take you through some adjustments that you can

make to the 'rules' for relaxing your sleep restriction, and improving your sleep efficiency. These will help to improve your sleep efficiency in a personalised way and work towards our goal of getting the amount of sleep you actually need.

Night owls and morning larks

We have spoken before about what we call chronotype. Most people are neither extreme larks nor owls. However, if you are an evening person, it may be better for you to select a later sleep window from Figure 27, and if you are a morning person an early window may be more suitable. Remember, night owls don't feel sleepy till later than morning larks.

Don't overdo it

I think there is a good chance that you will be worried by the rise time and threshold time you arrived at. It is likely that you will feel that it is very early to get up, or that it seems very late to stay up. Maybe you think that both will be a major problem. So, I want to make sure that you don't overdo things. I don't want you to become sleep deprived. If your total hours of sleep is fewer than 5 hours, I want you to work out your threshold time based on a *minimum of 5 hours in bed*. That's precisely why Figure 27 doesn't have sleep window options lower than 5 hours. Also, I often say to my patients who have a chronic health condition or a psychiatric illness to use a 6-hour minimum window. Please use your judgement and remember that I am trying to help you get a new and consistent sleep pattern going, but I don't want you to push yourself too far. Remember that a brief nap helps to address sleepiness, so if following sleep restriction is making you sleepy, as well as having a minimum window, you can use naps to keep you safe.

Increasing your sleep window based on progress

Although the restriction on your sleep window will be tight at the beginning, and you may not feel you are getting enough sleep, I don't expect that you will get stuck with that pattern. Indeed, you will end up getting more sleep because, once your pattern adjusts, you can begin to lengthen the amount of time you spend in bed. At first, the idea is that by restricting the amount of time you spend in bed you will be able to sleep right through. Instead of having bits of sleep, I want to see it all squashed together. But then we can let it grow a bit bigger, hopefully to the amount you would like . . . or at least to the amount you need.

Your guide here, again, is your sleep efficiency. Once you are sleeping 85-90 per cent of the time you are in bed (threshold time to rising time) for one full week, you can increase your time in bed by 15 minutes for the next week, by either going to bed 15 minutes earlier or staying in bed 15 minutes later in the morning. After trying that out for the next week, you can check if you still make it to 85-90 per cent. If you do, then you can increase your sleep window by another 15 minutes. The example of Ella in Box 17 illustrates how this works.

BOX 17: INCREASING YOUR SLEEP WINDOW BASED ON INCREASES IN SLEEP EFFICIENCY

Ella has been following a 6-hour sleep window and is now managing to sleep an average of 5½ hours per night. When she does the arithmetic, her sleep efficiency is now over 90 per cent $(5.5/6) \times 100 = 91.7$ per cent. So, during the next week she can increase her sleep window to 6 hours and 15 minutes. She can either set her alarm for 15 minutes later, or she can go to bed 15 minutes earlier. She cannot do both. This new schedule can then be followed for a further week to see if she is able to sleep even longer.

But please note you must be very strict and try not to go above 15 minutes per week! You can make these adjustments several times perhaps, but you will come to the point when you are in fact sleeping as much as you need. At that point, trying to spend longer in bed will not give you any more sleep and you have achieved your established pattern!

Compressing your sleep as an option

I think the method I have suggested for improving your sleep efficiency is the best one. However, there is one other option for you to consider, if you have been finding the sleep restriction approach too difficult. This alternative is called sleep compression. What you do here is reduce the amount of time you spend in bed by pressing in on your time in bed at both ends. By staying up a bit later and rising a bit earlier you can squeeze out some wakeful time in bed and increase your sleep efficiency. You can decide how much compression to use, but you need to make it enough to have some effect. You can make that decision based on your sleep efficiency (Figure 25). If your sleep efficiency starting point is low, then you will need to squeeze quite a bit. Just as with the restriction method, you can adjust the compression depending on how your sleep efficiency responds. Again, I think that intervals of 15 minutes are a good gauge for adjustment.

Summary of behavioural therapeutics for insomnia

This brings us to the end of this section of the programme, and I want to pull things together before you move on.

Strengthening your bed–sleep connection and improving your sleep efficiency can go hand in hand. Look back at Figure 22 as a reminder, but also look at Box 18 where I have summarised the behavioural elements for you.

BOX 18: PUTTING YOUR BEHAVIOURAL THERAPEUTICS PROGRAMME TOGETHER

1. Work out the amount of sleep you are getting and your sleep efficiency starting point. (Are you using diary and other data to inform your thinking?)

---

2. Stay up until your threshold time. (When is that? How are you going to use the extra time in the evening?)

3. Go to bed and lie down only when you feel sleepy tired. (What are your signs of sleepiness?)

4. Strengthen the bed–sleep connection. (What changes are you going to have to make?)

5. If you do not get to sleep, follow the quarter of an hour rule. (What exactly will you do when you get up? What preparations do you need to make before you even go to bed?)

6. If you still cannot fall asleep, repeat step 5. (What exactly will you do?)

7. If you wake during the night, repeat steps 5 and 6. (What exactly will you do?)

8. Get up in the morning at your fixed rising time. (How will you make sure?)

9. Do not nap during the day or evening, right up to your threshold time, unless sleepiness would be dangerous. (How are you going to avoid napping?)

10. Follow this programme seven days/nights a week. (How will you manage this?)

11. Use data like your sleep efficiency calculations to adjust the programme. (How will you make sure to keep completing your diary?)

12. Stay motivated to stick to the programme. (How are you going to do that?)

You will see that I have added some questions to help you think about each instruction in practical terms. I suggest that you note down your answers to each of these questions, and that you problem-solve any that are likely to pose a particular difficulty. If you have a partner or there are others in the house with you, it can be a good idea to discuss these solutions with them. I would remind you again about the importance of your sleep diary because it is very valuable in putting behavioural therapeutics into place and making the adjustments you need to make.

It feels like surgery!

I did mention that establishing your new sleep pattern was the most difficult part of CBT (Table 6), and now you probably see why! I know that the behavioural part is going to be tough for you, and that's why I sometimes call it the 'surgical option'. It is a bit like cutting out an old and malfunctioning part and implanting a working replacement! That's also why I told you that the behavioural part of CBT can be the most effective.

I emphasised the importance of staying motivated in Box 18 precisely because I know that these changes can be difficult to put into practice, and they can be even harder to keep going. You may find that the first few nights are not too bad and that you manage without difficulty. However, you will definitely be tempted at times, for example, to go to bed before your threshold time, to forego the quarter-of-an-hour rule, or to sleep in on the weekend. It is at times like these that you have to make that extra effort and stick to your new sleep schedule.

You have to remember that this insomnia is a tough problem to overcome, and that if the CBT programme is to work for you, you have to follow it the way it was designed. I have to say that it is only by maintaining the changes you have put in place that your sleep pattern can be improved. So, it is important that negative thoughts such as 'I am never going to get a good night's sleep' are replaced with more positive ones such as 'This problem is hard to break, but I am going to keep on following this programme because it has been shown to be effective for people like me.' *Keeping motivated* is the key to achieving permanent changes in your sleep pattern.

The diagram I produced for you in Chapter 6 (Figure 17) showed you the process of making changes when it is hard to do so. Have another look at that now and re-read that earlier section. Your motivation will come and go; that is to be expected. Relapses will occur some nights when you just can't follow the plan. These are times when you will experience a strong feeling of disappointment in yourself and think that there is no point trying again. Please don't let relapses discourage you. They are normal. The best thing to do is to get right back on course. I honestly think you may never have a better chance to sort out your sleep problems.

11

Reducing Your Arousal – Relaxation Therapeutics

Introduction

The relevance of relaxation therapeutics to overcoming insomnia lies in the fact that it is difficult to be stressed and relaxed at the same time. This may sound rather obvious; but think about it for a moment. If you are feeling relaxed, or know how to get yourself relaxed, the stress response has nothing to 'grab on to', and so your level of arousal is likely to decline rather than escalate. This can really help where sleep is concerned. If you are too wound up to sleep, especially if that tension feels very real and physical, then the relaxation approach could be exactly what you need.

You may be already thinking along these lines and have immediately turned to this chapter, after considering your options in Table 6. Alternatively, relaxation may be an approach that you want to add to the other cognitive or behavioural approaches that you have started. Either way, I think you will find help here. Importantly, I know that most people feel they have tried various forms of relaxation before, and you might be thinking that this won't work.

Well, let's see about that. I think you could be surprised about the difference being relaxed about your sleep can make! The aim of this chapter then is *to help you reduce your level of arousal so that you can sleep more easily.*

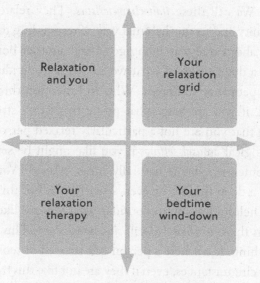

Figure 28: Components of relaxation

As you can see in Figure 28, I want to cover four main areas with you as we think through how to get you more relaxed. First, we will take a look at you as a person. Is your general approach to life relaxed, or not? Then we will review what I call your relaxation grid; the ways in which you typically relax. Next, we will explore your bedtime wind-down routine to see how sleep friendly it is. Finally, I will teach you an effective relaxation therapy that my patients have found to be very helpful.

Relaxation and you

So, let's start with you! Everyone is different. Some people are naturally relaxed, 'chilled', 'laid back' or whatever term you might use, whilst others are more tense or serious by nature. We call these *trait characteristics*. They relate to our personality and to our habitual way of responding to things. It's not about one way being good and another being bad. It's just a description of what we are like as individuals, and as I say people are different. Why do I mention this?

Well, if you are somewhat prone to getting stressed, it may be that you are not a particularly relaxed person. Your physiological *arousal settings* if you like might be set higher than someone who is naturally more relaxed. You might also be a deep thinker or even a worrier. All of this is OK, but it's helpful for you to consider what you are like.

Then there is what we call *situational stress*. This is a different thing. It is where a person gets stressed or tense under certain circumstances, even if they are not like this by nature. It is a *stress reaction* to particular events. In psychology, we call the symptoms you experience at these times *state characteristics* because they reflect how you feel at a given moment. Of course, it is likely that trait and state factors come together when a person with a tendency to trait arousal reacts more strongly to a given situation.

I hope you can see the relevance of this to difficulties getting to sleep or getting back to sleep if you waken up. Your level of arousal may be too high to get to sleep; and you may become even more aroused in that situation when you realise that you can't sleep. It is well worth thinking through what you are like and how you react to things, and even discussing it with someone you trust. It could help explain some of your struggles with sleep. Even knowing some of this may help with the RAPIDLY formulation and your 'good enough' explanation that we spoke about before (Figure 18; and Box 4). It could also help you to see why a more relaxed approach might work for you.

Your relaxation grid

Let's think next about the *importance* of relaxation. I'm sure most people would say that being able to relax is a good thing, but by our behaviour it isn't always obvious that we *value* relaxation. That's perhaps why we don't spend enough time prioritising and enjoying activities that bring us relaxation.

Our lives can be so full of the words *should, shouldn't, must* and *mustn't* that we don't give ourselves permission to relax! We might even feel that we *shouldn't* just sit and relax for a while, especially when there are '*things that need to be done*'. Does any of this sound familiar? If so, you could try to learn the value of relaxing. We're simply not designed to be on the go 24 hours a day, or to treat sleep as just a break from constant activity. We can work on valuing relaxation and bringing it more into our lives by using a simple relaxation grid.

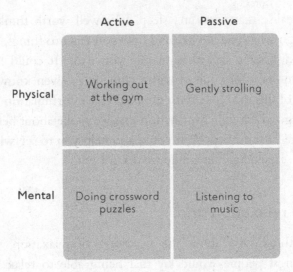

Figure 29: Your relaxation grid

As you can see in Figure 29, there are really four types of *relaxation*. There is the relaxation that we get from *active* pursuits: 'high energy' relaxation, if you like, where we burn up physical and mental stress. Then there is more *passive* relaxation, which is like 'letting go' rather than burning up. Let's consider this in a little more detail.

Sometimes people relax by 'active physical' means like exercise (say working out in the gym), and others use an 'active mental' approach, and relax by keeping their minds rather than their bodies busy (like researching their family history or doing puzzles). It is a little bit harder to use passive (gentle and more inactive) ways of relaxing, but there are good examples. As you can see, going for a stroll fits into the 'passive physical' box, and listening to music or an easy read book could be ways to relax in a 'passive mental' way. All of these forms of relaxation are useful, and I think it would help you if you could think about what activities you could do in each of the *four boxes* in Figure 29. What tools do you already have in the relaxation toolbox? What skills do you still need to develop? How can you become a good all-rounder?

The passive, 'letting go' kind of skills are often the ones that people struggle with. If your immediate thought is *'I don't have time for that'* or if you are the kind of person who feels the need to be productive all the time, then allowing yourself to relax may be part of the problem. And that certainly doesn't help at night when it comes to sleep, which is all about *letting go*!

So, consider your relaxation grid carefully. Remember that being able to relax quickly is useful, so even 5 or 10 minutes here or there can be worthwhile. Try to have something that you can commit to in each of the boxes because having a good mix of different ways to relax is going to help you in general, and also to help you prepare for sleep.

Your bedtime wind-down

It is a completely ridiculous idea to expect that you will just fall into bed and fall asleep because you happen to believe it is 'bed-time'. OK, you are going to say that some people can! Well, maybe so. But on the other hand, *you* have got a sleep problem and they don't. And then again, maybe it is more common for people who sleep well to be good at winding down before bedtime.

This is why I am going to suggest that you should develop a *wind-down* routine starting at least 60–90 minutes before bed so that you can start relaxing and preparing for sleep. Your routine should include things like slowing down your work/activity and then stopping it. Yes, I mean stopping work and stopping any other activities that involve taking responsibility, fixing things, and solving problems. You can then have a relaxed hour or more to wind-down, before getting into the immediate pre-bed activities of locking up, brushing your teeth, putting your pyjamas on, setting your alarm clock, and so on. Your wind-down routine should be on the one hand carefully planned, but on the other hand should not be rigid or inflexible. I have provided you with a planner (Figure 30) that you can personalise to suit your own times and activities.

Just a few tips, then it is up to you to consider the detail. It is a good idea to have an actual deadline to mark the transition from busy-ness to relaxation. Why not put a reminder or notification in your calendar, and tell other people that you are in the wind-down mode? It can also help to have something specific that you always do at that notification time, like put the kettle on to have a drink and a light snack, take command of the TV controls to watch a favourite programme, or settle down on the sofa with your book. Whatever you choose, it comes to serve as a marker of change, and helps you develop a new habit from that time in the evening onwards. People often get over-concerned about exactly what they should or should not do in that wind-down period. They ask me 'is it OK to do . . . or . . .?' It seems to me that they are feeling vulnerable in case

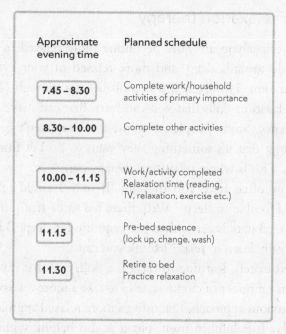

Approximate evening time	Planned schedule
7.45 – 8.30	Complete work/household activities of primary importance
8.30 – 10.00	Complete other activities
10.00 – 11.15	Work/activity completed Relaxation time (reading, TV, relaxation, exercise etc.)
11.15	Pre-bed sequence (lock up, change, wash)
11.30	Retire to bed Practice relaxation

Figure 30: An example of bedtime wind-down

they get it wrong. Let me remind you that you are not walking a tightrope to get your sleep routines right. That's not a relaxed approach! So, I tell them, and I say to you, that the important thing is that this period before retiring to bed should help you start unwinding. Do things that help you relax and let go. Experiment of course and find a good routine that works for you. This may be the one time of the day when you have some quality time for yourself, or that you can chat and enjoy time with your partner. Make this wind-down time special so that you look forward to it. It will then properly serve the purpose of helping you relax.

Your relaxation therapy

I hope that you are now becoming more relaxed in your attitude towards sleep, and more relaxed in your evening preparation. However, this is probably not enough. There are relaxation skills that you can learn that can make a big difference. Some people say to me that they aren't good at relaxing; that it's something they want to do but find difficult. This is where relaxation therapy comes in.

How often have you thought 'If only I could relax, I would be able to sleep'? Well, there has to be truth in that. A relaxed state is certainly a pre-requisite for sleep. But can you really learn to relax? I think you can.

Fortunately, learning to relax is a skill, one that can help you in a number of circumstances to take a more relaxed and less anxious approach. Practising a more relaxed approach in the day is helpful in itself, but it is also helpful with both technique and attitude at night. So how do you relax?

As I mentioned earlier, in my experience, people with insomnia often have difficulty with the *passive* approach to relaxation, the letting-go bit. It's so important with sleep that we learn to let it happen and not try to force it. I've decided, therefore, that I should give you a way of learning how to relax by letting go, using a technique that I use with my patients in my sleep clinic. The research evidence is that all relaxation methods have a similar effect, be they autogenic training, meditation, mindfulness, self-hypnosis or muscular relaxation.

The technique I use is called *progressive relaxation training* and it includes components from other relaxation procedures.

Progressive relaxation training involves exercises to tense and then relax the main muscle groups, which lead to decreases in muscle activity, blood pressure, and heart rate. It also includes help with breathing control and imagery (picturing) and awareness (autogenics) of your relaxation responses.

Here is the text of what I say to my patients when I am going through relaxation training with them. Giving you this is the easiest way I can think of to help you learn the technique. One suggestion is that you read the text out slowly and record it (once you are familiar with it). That would give you a recording that you could listen to, to guide your practice. If you do it properly the exercises should take 10–12 minutes.

Instructions for using progressive relaxation

These exercises are designed to help you relax. Relaxation is a skill which you can learn. It is just like any other skill, so don't be surprised if you find it takes practice, because that is how we learn skills. So do practise. Practise a couple of times a day, especially as you start to learn.

It is best to practise at a time when you know you won't be disturbed. The exercises will last between 10 and 12 minutes, so you will need at least that length of time set aside. When you do your relaxation exercises in your bed you will be able to listen to the recording there, if you have made one. But after a while you will have learned what to do and you will be able to follow the exercises in your own mind.

Progressive relaxation training exercise

Settle yourself down. Lie down with your hands and arms by your sides; have your eyes closed. That's good.

We will start by just thinking about your breathing. Your breathing can help you relax; the more deep and relaxed it is, the better you will feel and the more in control you will feel. So, begin by taking some slow regular breaths. Do that now. Breathe in fully, fill up your lungs fully; breathe in, hold your breath for a few seconds now, and let go, breathe out . . . Do that again, another deep breath, filling your lungs fully when you breathe in, hold it . . . and relax, breathe out. Continue in your own time, noticing that each time you breathe in the muscles in your chest tighten up, and as you breathe out there is a sense of letting go. You can think the word 'relax' each time you breathe out. This will remind you that breathing out helps you relax. It will also help you use this word to tell yourself to relax whenever you need to. You will find that your body will begin to respond. Breathing slowly, comfortably, regularly, and deeply; thinking the word 'relax' every time you breathe out; enjoying just lying still and having these moments to relax, concentrating on the exercises.

Now I'd like you to turn your attention to your arms and hands. I'd like you to create some tension in your hands and arms by pressing your fingers into the palms of your hands and making fists. Do that with both hands now. Feel the tension in your hands, feel the tension in your fingers and your wrists, feel the tension in your forearms. Notice what it is like. Keep it going . . . and now relax. Let those hands flop. Let them do whatever they want to do; just let them relax. Notice the difference that's taken place between tension and relaxation. Breathing slowly and deeply, you will find that your fingers will just straighten out and flop, and your hands and arms will feel more relaxed. Allow them to sink into the couch or into the bed; just allow your arms to be heavy. Breathing slowly and deeply, thinking the word 'relax' each time you breathe out, and finding that your hands and arms just relax more and more and more. Your arms and your hands are so heavy and rested. It's almost as if you couldn't be bothered moving them. Just because you have let go of the energy and tension that was in the muscles there. Breathing slowly and deeply, both your hands, both your arms, heavy and rested. Let go of the energy and tension that was in the muscles there, breathing slowly and deeply. Both your hands, both your arms, heavy and rested and relaxed.

I'd like you to turn your attention now to your neck and shoulders. Again, we're going to get your neck and shoulders into a state of relaxation following some tension we're going to introduce. I'd like you to do that by pulling your shoulders up towards your ears. Now, do that; pull your shoulders up towards your ears. Feel the tension across the back of your neck, across the top of your back and in your shoulders. Feel the tension, keep it going not so much that it's sore, but keep it constant. Feel it, and now let go . . . relax; go back to breathing slowly and deeply. Let that tension drain away, let it go. Breathe deeply, and as you do so, notice that the tension, almost like a stream, drains away from your neck, across your shoulders, down the upper part of your arms, down the lower part of your arms and out through your fingertips. Draining out and leaving a sense of warmth and relaxation deep in your muscles. Breathing slowly and deeply and allowing that to take place. Just let the tension go. If it doesn't seem to go, don't force it, it will go itself. Be confident about that. Just breathe slowly and deeply and allow yourself to be relaxed; remembering to think the word 'relax' each time you breathe out. Using that word 'relax' to focus on the sense of relaxation that you get, using the word 'relax' to remind you of the success you are having in relaxing your body.

I'd like you to concentrate now on your face, and on your jaw, and on your forehead. I'd like you to create some tension in these parts of your body by doing two things together at the same time. These things are to screw up your eyes really tightly and bite your teeth together. Do these things together now. Bite your teeth together; feel the tension in your jaw. Screw up your eyes; feel the tension all around your eyes, in your forehead, in your cheeks, throughout your face, wherever there is tension. Now keep it going . . . and relax; breathing in through your nose and out through your mouth, slowly and deeply. Notice how your forehead smoothes out and then your eyelids and your cheeks. Allow your jaw to hang slightly open. Allow your whole head to feel heavy and to sink into the pillow; breathing slowly and deeply. Allow there to be a spread of relaxation across the surface of your face and into all those muscles in your face. Allow your eyelids to feel heavy and comfortable, your jaw and your whole head; breathing slowly and deeply, enjoying the relaxation which you feel in your body. Relax each time you breathe out. Relax just that little bit more each time you breathe out.

Concentrating now on your legs and feet, I want you to create some tension here by doing two things at the same time; and these things are to press the backs of your legs downwards and to pull your toes back towards your head. Do these things together now. Create the tension in your legs, press the backs of your legs downwards and pull your toes back towards your head. Feel the tension in your feet, in your toes, in your ankles, in the muscles in your legs. Feel what it is like. Don't overdo it; just notice what it is like

. . . hold it . . . and now relax. Breathing slowly and deeply once more; just allow your feet to flop any old way. Thinking the word 'relax' each time you breathe out. Allow the muscles to give up their energy, give up their tension. Let it go, breathing slowly and deeply. Notice how your feet just want to flop to the side. Notice how your legs feel heavy as if you couldn't be bothered moving them. Heavy and comfortable and rested and relaxed. Just that little bit more relaxed each time you breathe out.

Be thinking about your whole body now; supported by the bed or chair, sinking into it, but supported by it. You've let go the tension throughout your body. Your body feels rested, comfortable. Enjoy each deep breath you take. Just use these few moments now to think about any part of your body that doesn't feel quite so rested and allow the tension to go. It will go. Breathe slowly and deeply; thinking the word 'relax' each time you breathe out. Just let any remaining tension drain away; from your hands, your arms, your neck and your back. Heavy and rested, comfortable and relaxed. From your face and your eyes, from your forehead; letting the muscles give up their energy. Like a stream of relaxation flowing over your whole body. Let your legs and feet feel relaxed; sinking into the bed. Breathing slowly and deeply.

In a few moments, the exercises will be finished; but you can continue to relax. You may wish to repeat some of the exercises yourself and that is fine. You may wish to enjoy just continuing as you are. It's up to you . . . but continue to relax.

Personalising your relaxation therapy

I have mentioned a couple of ways in which you can personalise relaxation therapy, let me mention them again and then add some further thoughts. I have summarised them all in Box 19.

BOX 19: PERSONALISING YOUR RELAXATION THERAPY

1. Record your relaxation therapy using the script provided and use the recording to practise and learn the technique.
2. Set aside time to practise. Make it a priority in your day-to-day activities.
3. Personalise the content of the programme, according to your needs.
4. Consider linking relaxation with imagery training or mindfulness for a more extended therapy session.

First, you can make a recording of the therapy. It might take you a few tries to get it right, but I think it is worth the effort. It's so much easier to listen and to respond and follow rather than having to read it each time to yourself!

Second, you can also personalise your practice. There's no set way to do this, but the emphasis should be on finding time to develop skills in relaxing, and in learning the therapy so that you can do it without needing to listen to the replay. Practice as they say makes perfect, so be prepared to put in a bit of time. The more you know what you are doing, the more useful it will be to switch into the relaxed mode in bed.

Third, some people find parts of the programme difficult. That could be the case for example if you have been experiencing pain in part of your body, or if you have some movement difficulties. You might also be uncomfortable lying in a certain position, for example if you are pregnant, or 10–12 minutes might not be the best amount of time. Some people prefer shorter, some longer. I want you to feel free to adapt the programme to one that works for you. For example, you could limit the tension–release cycles and concentrate more on giving yourself instructions to 'let go'. You could also concentrate more on allowing yourself to relax as you breathe out and encouraging yourself to feel heavy and rested. These alterations to relaxation therapy are similar to what happens in autogenic training and in the 'body scan' technique that is sometimes used in mindfulness. They all have the same end point in allowing you to let go.

Fourth, it can be helpful to extend your relaxation therapy by using imagery training or mindfulness. Look back at the techniques I introduced in the chapter on cognitive therapeutics. I think you will see how these could dovetail with the relaxation routine. I have also suggested that incorporating relaxation into your lifestyle is a healthy option!

Finally, remember that your relaxation is not meant to put you to sleep. The exercises are useful to help prepare you for sleep, so that a relaxed you can fall asleep naturally! Try to avoid asking yourself the question 'am I sleepy?', stop monitoring yourself all the time, and just enjoy relaxing.

Summary of relaxation therapeutics for insomnia

So, in concluding this section on relaxation therapeutics, let's try to bring things together. Your bedtime wind-down and pre-bed routine should encourage you to switch off from the day and to relax in preparation for sleep. The progressive relaxation training is there to help you relax even more. Here is what I mean, summarised in Box 20.

BOX 20: YOUR RELAXATION THERAPEUTICS SUMMARY

- Know and accept yourself. Try to understand what relaxation means to you and how it might help you.
- Consider how to introduce relaxation opportunities into your life. Be prepared to try new approaches.
- Establish a wind-down routine in the second half of the evening. Set a deadline for work/activity, 90 minutes before bed.
- Learn progressive relaxation therapy as a skill. Personalise it to your needs.

12

Improving Your Sleep Hygiene

Introduction

Earlier in Part Three, and as you saw in Table 6, I explained that this chapter on sleep hygiene, and the following one on improving your sleep knowledge, are there to support your therapy. If I was trying to provide you with a meal these elements would not be a main course! I place much greater emphasis on the cognitive, behavioural and relaxation therapeutics parts of CBT because they will help you most to overcome your insomnia. Having said that, it is definitely worth reviewing your sleep hygiene, so feel free to dip into this chapter whenever you think it may be helpful.

What is *sleep hygiene*?! I agree it is a strange term, and not one I particularly like! However, it is increasingly being used, so we are kind of stuck with it now. On the positive side it conveys the idea of the 'sleep basics': what anyone could do to tidy up their sleep preparation, if you like. Sleep hygiene refers to things about your lifestyle and your preparation for bed that might be changed to improve your sleep health. Sometimes there may be a simple solution to a sleep problem, such as stopping drinking excessive amounts of coffee. However, for most people it is more about making the most of all of the good sleep hygiene practices to make sure that you are better prepared for sleep.

Sleep hygiene can be split into two parts. First, how your lifestyle affects your sleep, and second, how you can ensure your bedroom environment supports good sleep. We will take these two areas in turn, and then go on to consider the very important matter of relaxation. The purpose of this chapter then is to *develop a lifestyle that supports good sleep and to create a sleep-friendly bedroom.*

Good lifestyle, good sleep?

The main lifestyle factors known to have an effect on sleep are: caffeine, nicotine, alcohol, diet and exercise. I would like to give you some recommendations about each of these.

Caffeine

Caffeine is a type of drug called a stimulant. This means that it perks you up by having a stimulating effect on your nervous system. Too much caffeine is very good at keeping you awake!

Most people know that caffeine is found in coffee and tea, but many other products also contain caffeine. For example, cocoa, chocolate bars, soft drinks like sodas and energy drinks, some alcohol products and some medicines you can buy at the store for headaches and to help you lose weight. Because caffeine is found in so many different products, I have a suggestion – try this little exercise. Have a rummage in your kitchen cupboards, in your refrigerator and in your medicine cabinet. See how many products you can find that have caffeine listed on them as an ingredient. You can use Table 13 to keep a note as you go along.

I suggest that you make a special point of checking the labels on things you might eat or drink in the evening and before bedtime. Caffeine's effects can last for many hours and it is a good idea not to have any caffeine in the 4 hours before bedtime.

If you would like to cut down on caffeine, or cut out caffeine altogether, you can try switching to caffeine-free drinks such as decaffeinated tea or coffee, herbal tea or caffeine-free cola. Please note that some people who are used to drinking caffeinated beverages on a daily basis experience headaches for the first few days of not drinking them. This is like a withdrawal effect, but it disappears quickly after a couple of days.

Nicotine

Nicotine, which is found in cigarettes and other tobacco products, is also a stimulant drug and has similar effects to caffeine on sleep. Although many people say that they find that smoking is relaxing, the overall effect of nicotine on the body's central nervous system is that of stimulation. What this means is that nicotine will make it harder to fall asleep and harder to stay asleep.

Table 13: Caffeine products that you use

Products in the kitchen containing caffeine	Products elsewhere in the house/at work/ when dining out containing caffeine

These days of course many people are not smoking tobacco but are using e-cigarettes or 'vaping' instead. It is important to think this through because the main health benefit of vaping over tobacco smoking is the reduction or elimination of carcinogens found in tar. However, most vaping devices are simply electronic nicotine delivery systems, unless you use one that is nicotine free.

So, if you do smoke or vape, I recommend that you try and cut down in the evening before you go to bed, and that you try not to smoke if you wake up in the middle of the night. You need to consider the possibility that you wake up with a craving for nicotine and that this has become part of your smoking habit. I know all this is easier said than done, but it could be important.

Alcohol

Alcohol, unlike caffeine and nicotine, is a depressant drug. Normally, depressants should help us sleep, but it has been found that even a moderate amount of alcohol in the evening can actually have a disruptive effect on sleep.

Alcohol may help you to fall into a deep sleep at the beginning of the night. In this sense it is an effective hypnotic drug. However, as the alcohol gets absorbed into your body, mild withdrawal symptoms occur that may be sufficient to wake you up or put you into a lighter form of sleep. Alcohol-induced sleep therefore is not normal sleep and it can cause disturbed dreams. Alcohol can also make you dehydrated so you may wake up thirsty in the middle of the night and need to go to the toilet more often than usual. I should also mention that alcohol acts as a muscle relaxant and that can cause your breathing in sleep to be more laboured, and you may snore heavily.

For people with persistent insomnia, the use of alcohol in an effort to promote sleep is particularly unwise because it can encourage dependence. I recommend that you avoid drinking alcohol from 4 hours before bedtime. Sorry that I cannot really support the idea of a 'nightcap'!

Diet

Hunger can cause wakefulness. That is why a light snack an hour or two before bedtime can help us sleep. On the other hand, going to bed too full can also cause wakefulness. Our bodies are busy digesting the food, and this interferes with sleep.

People often ask me about milk and other dairy products and whether they promote sleep. There are many old beliefs about having a warm milky drink before bed to help you fall off to sleep. The evidence on milk products improving the quality of a person's sleep however is very doubtful. I guess what we can say with some certainty, though, is that it is preferable to caffeinated coffee or tea.

The same can be said of many other food or dietary products that are sold as sleep-promoting. Products containing tryptophan for example often try to have a credible story written behind them, but this is more marketing than science. The evidence is scarce, and I don't think there is a meaningful effect that you would notice, apart perhaps from the placebo effect. Such products are certainly not treatments for insomnia.

It is probably wise also to avoid snacking if you wake up in the night, as your body may come to expect food at this time. If you do snack at night, then you run the risk of continuing to wake up to satisfy your hunger. A glass of water at the side of the bed is a good idea because a few sips help freshen the mouth and take the edge off your thirst, without causing you to have to run to the bathroom.

Weight changes can also have some effect upon sleep. Too much weight loss over a short time period may lead to short, broken-up sleep. If you are trying to lose weight, I suggest that you aim to lose no more than a pound or two per week, and that you stick to your programme of weight reduction until you achieve your target weight. Heavier people are more likely to snore, which can disrupt sleep both for themselves and others . . . and losing weight can reduce snoring.

In general, healthy people are better sleepers, so managing your diet to maintain a healthy weight, and to reduce your body fat, is by far the best advice I can give you about the relationship between diet and sleep.

Exercise

People who are physically fit have a better quality of sleep, so a good way to promote sleep is to get fit by exercising at least three times a week for 20–30 minutes. The type of exercise you do really depends on what kind of activities you enjoy. It is recommended, however, that in order to get fit and stay fit, you should take up exercise that gets your heart pumping. Walking, swimming, cycling, skating, football, squash, badminton and aerobics are just a few of the many activities that do this. If you are unsure about exercising, please talk to your doctor before starting an exercise programme.

Although being fit is beneficial to sleep, there is mixed evidence about what happens when you take strenuous exercise before bedtime. In some people, exercise taken late on 'wakes up' the nervous system and can lead to problems falling asleep and problems staying asleep. Even exercise in the evening may have these unwanted effects. On the other hand, it is definitely a good thing to have exercise as part of your daily routine and some people may find that exercise acts as a circuit-breaker before they settle down to relax for the evening. I suggest that you experiment a bit with the level and timing of your exercise and see what works best for you.

I would certainly advise against exercising for the wrong reasons. The idea that some people have of going out before bed to exhaust themselves so that they can fall into a sound sleep is not a good one! I would say plan your exercise to become fit and to stay healthy. Don't use exercise as a weapon against insomnia.

Table 14: Sleep hygiene changes in my lifestyle

Caffeine
Nicotine
Alcohol
Diet
Exercise

Let's have a pause for thought at this point. Do you think that your lifestyle could be improved to help you sleep? Write down any decisions you have made about each of these lifestyle areas in Table 14. You can keep coming back to your decisions to see if you have carried them through!

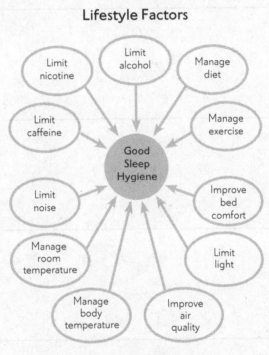

Lifestyle Factors

Limit nicotine

Limit alcohol

Manage diet

Limit caffeine

Manage exercise

Good Sleep Hygiene

Limit noise

Improve bed comfort

Manage room temperature

Limit light

Manage body temperature

Improve air quality

Bedroom Factors

Figure 31: Sleep hygiene factors to improve your sleep health

A sleep-friendly bedroom?

As you know there are two parts to sleep hygiene. You will see them illustrated in Figure 31, and so far, we have covered the top section on lifestyle. Now I want to help you think in the lower panel of Figure 31, about the bedroom, and ways of ensuring it is sleep-friendly. We are going to consider noise levels, room temperature, the quality of the air in the bedroom, lighting levels, and the comfort of the mattress and pillows to see if these might influence our sleep.

Noise

You will not be surprised to learn that noise can disrupt sleep. Unexpected and sudden noises, if loud enough, will wake most people either from the gentle reverie of the just-about-asleep stage, or even from deep sleep. The cry of a baby, the sound of a telephone ringing, a car horn and, of course, an alarm clock are all examples of these kinds of sounds. Some sounds are designed to attract our attention, like your morning alarm or your baby needing to be fed, and we become sensitised to these so that we hear and respond to them even when we are asleep.

However, we do also know that people can get used to noises after a while, although some folks may be better at this than others. For example, people who live in houses close to railway tracks seem to adapt to the sounds of passing trains. Also, most people get used to noise that is continuous, such as a ticking clock, or even a partner's snoring! Nevertheless, it can be that even if people do not actually wake up in response to noises, their sleep may be affected as a result of brief transitions from deeper to lighter forms of sleep.

Well, what about you? Try to figure out any noises in your home environment that may be interfering with your sleep and do what you can about them. Sleeping with earplugs may or may not be the answer for you. If you are troubled by outside noises, wearing earplugs may just cause you to listen in to your own inner sounds, like your breathing. But you could experiment and find out. There are a lot of noise reduction products that are marketed to help you sleep so there is plenty of choice. However, I wouldn't spend too much because the evidence for them is very limited, and they are likely not any better than simple earplugs. Probably you will find that distraction techniques, like relaxation exercises, are more helpful rather than getting too preoccupied with something you can't easily change and probably don't need to. Very few patients with insomnia think noise is the cause of their sleeping difficulty.

Room temperature

Extreme temperatures at either end of the range can affect our sleep. A room that is too hot (more than 24°C) can cause us to have restless body movements during sleep, and more night-time wakings. On the other hand, a room that is too cold (less than 12°C) can make it difficult to get to sleep and also make us restless and unsettled. I would suggest that your ideal room temperature to help promote sleep is likely to be around 18°C. Why don't you try it out and see?

Buy a thermometer and experiment with the climate in your bedroom!

Body Temperature

People sometimes like to take a hot bath or a shower because they find it helps them to relax. You might think this must be a good thing. However, it may or may not help you to get to sleep. We know, for example, that poor sleepers often report feeling hotter than good sleepers. It is not a good idea to be too hot when you go to bed, so I recommend that you can best prepare your body for bed by taking your bath around one hour before bedtime, rather than immediately before retiring. If you wanted to you could make it part of your pre-bed routine (at least some nights!).

You can of course make some adjustments to your temperature by trying different types of bedcovers. Again, don't worry about experimenting.

Air quality

A stuffy room is likely to cause an uncomfortable sleep, while fresh air will promote sleep. I find that many people actually don't ventilate the bedroom, so this could be something to try. Why don't you open a window before going to bed, or adjust the flow of the air-conditioning to give you fresh clean air? The circulation of good-quality air is going to be helpful. Of course, you have to bear in mind the seasons. You may not want to leave a window too far open all night, especially in the winter. See what you can do to adjust that blend of temperature and air control to find what is right for you.

Lighting

Do you remember when I explained how natural light is a major controlling factor in the sleep-wake (circadian) rhythm? We are all familiar with a parent saying that their child can't get to sleep because it is still light outside, or the child waking up earlier (in the summer) because it is getting light earlier. We do the same ourselves!

Natural light, of course, normally penetrates into the bedroom, too – through the window! Don't miss the obvious. Your bedroom at home should not be too bright. A combination of summer nights or even strong street lighting and thin curtains is avoidable. I would go as far as to say that your bedroom should be almost completely dark once you have switched off the light. Not totally dark, because that may cause anxiety as well as being rather unnatural.

The simplest solution is to cover windows with thick curtains (black-out curtains), blinds or even a blanket during your sleep period. Some people find they can sleep well with a sleep mask on, although not everybody will find these comfortable. If you prefer to have a bit of light, try to keep it at a very low level, like a small lamp in the hallway with the door ajar very slightly, or a plug-in night-light of minimal wattage. In the section on behavioural therapeutics I talk a bit about having devices in the bedroom. Many of these also emit light, but the biggest problem with them is not the light stimulation but the habit of staying awake to read, communicate on social media and so on.

Bed, mattress and pillows

There are a lot of personal preferences when it comes to pillows and mattresses, so it is hard for me to give advice that will suit everyone. One thing that does strike me, though, is that we know that people with insomnia sometimes sleep better in an unfamiliar environment. As mentioned earlier, this may be because they don't expect to sleep, so they don't worry about it quite so much. It may be because the triggers to poor sleep – all the associations with nights spent tossing and turning – are left back at home. But another simple possibility is that other beds suit their sleep needs better than their beds at home.

Could any of this apply to you? For example, beds in hotels are often larger and have firmer mattresses than domestic beds. Remember, too, that beds and mattresses of different qualities have differing life spans. A bed can be one of those things that what you pay for is what you get. You can experiment a bit, though. For example, if you have a soft mattress you can make it firmer by placing a board underneath it. But if you can feel the springs it is certainly time to buy a new one! You may also wish to try switching beds if there are others in your home, to see if you can find the level of comfort you need before purchasing. And salespeople in stores can actually be quite helpful.

There is no real standard for pillows. What people prefer and find most suitable depends a lot on personal taste. But don't make assumptions – be prepared to experiment again. It is also worth considering the amount of bed-covering you need for comfort, and the weight of covering that best suits you.

All this said, I wouldn't believe too much in the promotional materials around beds, mattresses, pillows and weighted blankets as a therapeutic option. All this is about consumer choice, not treatment. There is very little evidence that these are the problems causing insomnia in the first place.

Just as you did with lifestyle factors, I would like you now to use Table 15 to note down things that you think you need to consider about your bedroom and your sleep.

Take a final look at Figure 31 to ensure you get the bigger picture of lifestyle and bedroom factors that might affect your sleep, and make sure you work on anything that might make your sleep hygiene just a little bit better.

Table 15: Sleep hygiene changes in my bedroom

Noise
Temperature
Air quality
Lighting
Bed/mattress/pillows

13

Improving Your Sleep Knowledge

Introduction

As you know the navigational wheel (Figure 19) encourages you to find your best starting point for therapy in Chapter 9, 10 or 11. Nevertheless, your understanding about what sleep is and why sleep is important matters, so reading through this chapter on sleep knowledge may be helpful.

> *What we know and what we feel are not necessarily the same thing.*

I would encourage you to read this statement over a few times. It is very important. Let me give you an example. Phobias are interesting problems – we call them 'irrational fears' precisely because people with a phobia really *know* that the thing they fear is likely to be quite safe, but they do not *feel* that it is safe when they are faced with the situation. A person who is afraid of a spider knows when they focus on the facts that the spider is unlikely to hurt them. Can you see . . . that what we know (intellectually) and what we feel (emotionally) are not necessarily the same thing.

What has all this got to do with insomnia?

Well, in Part One you learned a lot about sleep, and about insomnia and its consequences. I would hope that by now you *know* more than you did before you started out. But can I ask you if you *feel* any differently about your sleep or any part of your sleep problem? Do you feel any differently about yourself, as a poor sleeper? For information to be of any real help to you it has to change not only the way you think but also the way you feel. In Part Two you began to assess your sleep pattern. Your sleep diary, for example, will have given you more detailed knowledge of how you are sleeping at present. What are you learning, how are you feeling about the potential to overcome your insomnia?

This chapter will give you more information about sleep, but it is also about encouraging you to have an open mind. Perhaps you need to form a fresh view about some things relating to sleep or insomnia? And to let the facts affect how you feel? I am also counting on the possibility that some of you reading the book will be thinking that you already knew almost everything I have said. But my comment applies to you, too, perhaps even more so. Read the statement above once more. You may already know a lot – my challenge to you is to use this information differently.

The purpose of this chapter therefore is to remind you about normal sleep and about sleep disorders and their effects, *and to use this information to make a difference to how you think and feel about your insomnia and about yourself.*

A sleep quiz

Let's see how much you remember from Part One. In Box 21 I have put together a quiz to test your knowledge. It is to get you thinking.

BOX 21: YOUR SLEEP QUIZ

1. People need less sleep in later life.   True/False

2. We tend to sleep better as the night goes on.   True/False

3. We should try to make up for all our lost sleep on subsequent nights.   True/False

4. Dreaming a lot is usually a sign of emotional upset.   True/False

5. Sleep is important for our memory.   True/False

6. The more sleep we can get, the better we will feel the next day.   True/False

7. Feeling irritable during the day probably means our sleep quality is poor.   True/False

---

8. Most adults sleep 7–8 hours at night.   True/False

9. There is really no such thing as 'deep sleep'.   True/False

10. Daytime tiredness may be an important sign of a sleep disorder.   True/False

11. Sleep problems usually pass away quite quickly.   True/False

12. Most people don't cope very well after a bad night's sleep.   True/False

13. Sleeping pills are addictive.   True/False

14. Taking a nap should be avoided if at all possible.   True/False

15. Life changes can trigger insomnia.   True/False

16. Some people seem to be able to do without sleep.   True/False

17. Insomnia causes depression and depression causes insomnia   True/False

18. I'd be better just giving up because I've tried it all before.   True/False

There are two ways you could do this. One possibility is that you just glance down the items starting at the first question, think to yourself 'True' or 'False', make a decision and then move on to the second question, and so on. That's fine. The other possibility, however, is to take some time to consider each answer. Jot down a few notes . . . weighing up the pros and cons for both true and false. I think you would get more out of doing it this second way, but it's up to you.

OK – now I will take you through my answers. Some of the statements were a bit tricky, I think, because it is not always a straightforward choice!

Quiz answers

<u>1. People need less sleep in later life</u>
The amount we sleep very much changes throughout our life cycle. The newborn baby might sleep for more than 18 hours, waking only to be fed; most infants and young children sleep from the early evening through to morning, as well as sometimes having naps in the daytime. 'Deep' sleep and 'dreaming' sleep are particularly plentiful in these early years because these types of sleep are associated with physical and mental development. At the opposite end of the age spectrum, older adults who are not using as much energy or discovering as much new information, have less stage 3, slow wave sleep. Older adults, in fact, tend to sleep less at night than younger adults, and can have more broken sleep, especially in the second half of the night. Of course, they may 'make up' for this to some extent by napping. It

is important to recognise that some of our sleep problems, for example 'lighter' sleep as we get older, are just normal changes. Changes like this can sometimes be very hard to accept. In short, the answer to this first point is TRUE.

Now this first quiz question is probably an example of something you already knew. But let me pose an important challenge to you: have you really adjusted your *expectations* of your sleep as you have grown older? Just because you know in your head that your sleep is likely to be more fragmented and that you may have less sleep at night, doesn't mean that you have accepted that change and are feeling OK about it.

Perhaps you have never thought of making any conscious decision about adjusting your sleep habits. But things do change. Not everyone still fits into their bridal gown or their wedding suit. Do you remember as a child, when you were gradually allowed to stay up a bit later . . . then later still? Those changes in bedtime pattern probably just reflected your sleep requirement at that age and stage of your life. This may be a good time to stop and think if adjustments might be appropriate again. You see, one major problem with insomnia is that we may overcompensate for our sleeplessness by spend-ing longer in bed – to try to catch up on more sleep. The problem is we can then end up with more frustration, simply because we are in bed for too long, compared with our ability to sleep. You maybe know about this vicious circle already!

2. We tend to sleep better as the night goes on

Don't we just love to get into a deep sleep? It might be nice to think of the night's journey in sleep as one big, deep valley with a flat bottom. That we gradually descend down the slopes from wakefulness into the fertile and expansive plain of deep sleep, and that, with the coming of the morning, we slowly rise up the other side to wakefulness once more. But it's not like that at all. Throughout the night we have different types of sleep. Some of it is 'lighter', some 'deeper', and some is REM sleep when we do most of our dreaming. We cycle through these stages each night. We have several sets of valleys and summits to negotiate on the night's journey. In fact, we have our deepest sleep very early on, and are pretty much done with deep sleep after the first couple of hours of the night! So, the answer here is undoubtedly FALSE.

But don't take this as bad news! What it means is that nature has organised things in such a way that even if our sleep is short in duration, we get the biggest payback out of the early sleep episodes, whenever we actually manage to get to sleep. These are the most restorative periods, and that is why you can sometimes wake quite refreshed after just a couple of hours of sleep. It is also why you don't need to catch up on all your 'lost' sleep.

3. We should try to make up for all our lost sleep on subsequent nights

This is one of the tricky ones . . . but I've just hinted at the answer!

You may remember that I explained about 'sleep debt'? The idea being that during the day we build up sleep debt that is then repaid at night, allowing us to start ideally with a zero balance at the beginning of the next new day. There might seem to be a danger then for people with insomnia. Not sleeping well might mean that they don't pay off sufficient debt and end up being in long-term arrears! But fortunately, this is where the sleep-debt model actually breaks down. We do not need to repay sleep loss on an hour-for-hour basis. The best evidence we have suggests that we need to make up around one-third of our lost hours. Furthermore, the sleep we get on recovery nights may be deeper and more restorative. I would say, therefore, that the answer to this question is FALSE. We should *not* try to make up for all our lost sleep on subsequent nights. However, the social jetlag phenomenon is important. Try to make sure that you get enough sleep on weekdays, as well as catching up a bit on weekends. You do need to catch up on a good part of your sleep if you are running short – just not 100% of it!

This can be a challenge in insomnia because if you are constantly worrying about catching up you will find yourself trying all the harder to get to sleep, which as you know just gets you more stressed and keeps you awake. Or you may try to go to bed early the next night to catch up. This doesn't work well either in insomnia because you make the catch up night an even longer one when you already have problems sleeping through a normal night. Best plan is to overcome your insomnia!

4. Dreaming a lot is usually a sign of emotional upset
We have several spells of dreaming sleep during the night, although of course some people remember their dreams more than others. That's partly dependent on whether or

not you wake out of REM sleep or non-REM sleep, and partly just individual differences. It actually doesn't really matter all that much because you are having them in any case. Dreams are a normal part of our sleep whether or not we remember them! Remember that sleep is an important time for information processing and for emotional regulation. Dreams are just a little window into the workings of the brain showing that processing work is going on.

Coming back to the question, the answer is certainly FALSE – dreaming itself is not a sign of emotional upset. The content of our dreams is largely unimportant and not worth trying to interpret. It is possible that we dream more when we have a lot on our minds, and there are people who have recurring dreams of a nightmarish quality. Such dreams may have some root in unpleasant experiences or unpleasant memories. In threatening dreams that are associated with traumatic stress people can be helped by 'rescripting' techniques to make them less of a nightmare. This is best done with an experienced clinician. In general terms, however, dreaming should be regarded as a healthy experience that is simply a reflection of REM sleep. People may also dream more than usual during withdrawal periods from sleeping pills, and also in the latter part of the night if they have consumed a significant amount of alcohol. These are both temporary factors influencing dreaming sleep.

5. Sleep is important for our memory

Sleep is a time when a lot goes on! It is important to realise that sleep is not simply the absence of wakefulness; it is a time when a great deal of different kinds of activity occurs. This activity takes place both in our minds and in our bodies. So, although we switch off the lights when we go to bed, we are not switching ourselves off when we fall asleep! I think our brain is delighted to get busy during our night, doing so much of its important work while we are asleep.

Sleep is necessary for both physical and mental health. Tired muscles and bodies need rest for our energy sources to recover, but we must have sleep to generate cells to rebuild and repair tissue, and for our body chemistry such as our immune function to work properly. The harder our bodies work, the more we may find we need to sleep. The same is true for our minds. While we mostly stop taking in new information through our senses, our brains are really still on the job. Sleep gives the brain the space and time to sort out information about things that have happened during the day. What we have experienced and learned is processed even though we are not usually conscious of it, and memories are being stored. All this is part of the mystery of the sleep process – we simply can't do without it! There is no doubt that sleep is important for our memory, probably more important than wakefulness in fact; so, the answer to this statement is TRUE.

6. The more sleep we can get, the better we will feel the next day

Let me say first of all that there is no direct relationship between quantity of sleep and well-being. Although it may be possible for people who are good sleepers to sleep more than they actually need, there is little evidence that they benefit in the daytime from doing so, except that it is nice to have that choice! There are even some disadvantages associated with oversleeping, because doing so may strengthen what we call *sleep inertia*. This is the experience we have of emerging from sleep into daytime waking with a feeling of struggling to get going. Oversleeping can contribute to sleep inertia rather than feeling refreshed, so the idea that the more you sleep the better you will feel is a bit of a pipe dream!

However, this is one of the tricky questions, because if you are not getting enough sleep, getting more sleep will help you feel better during the day. The total amount of sleep that people in the general population obtain follows what is known as a *normal distribution*. In other words, it is just as normal to be a short sleeper (someone with a shorter sleep requirement) as it is to be a long sleeper (a person with a longer sleep requirement). All of that is fine, but if you are a short sleeper AND you have insomnia, then that can be a difficult mix. Because long sleepers don't generally feel any better than short sleepers, I would say the answer to this item is FALSE, but I might allow you to take a point if you were thinking of short sleep plus insomnia!

The most important thing is to establish your personal sleep requirement, and to try to obtain that on a regular basis from night to night.

7. Feeling irritable during the day probably means our sleep quality is poor

It is undoubtedly true that irritability can be associated with insomnia, but again this is one of those tricky ones, because there are, after all, many other reasons why we may become irritable during the day!

This is an example of what we call *attribution* or *beliefs.* We know that people who have insomnia will be likely to attribute experiences that they have in the daytime to having slept poorly, but that does not necessarily mean that the insomnia has actually caused these events. Poor sleep can definitely make us irritable, but I think on balance I would answer this one as FALSE, on the basis that irritability could equally well be associated with frustration at work, difficulty solving a problem, relationship difficulties, and so on. That is not, however, to deny the important relationship between night-time sleep and daytime mood.

I must confess I put this item in the quiz quite deliberately to help you to think through the whole issue of attribution. Think back to the statement 'What we know and what we feel are not necessarily the same thing.' It is important to evaluate your strength of feeling that irritability (or any other daytime symptom, such as tiredness) results directly from your insomnia. More than that, it is important to evaluate your belief in that particular association, over and against any other possible explanation. This process of evaluation will help you to make more accurate attributions. Then you will be in the strongest position to deal more effectively with the most likely causes of how you are feeling. So, for example, you may find that there are stressors at work that need some attention, as well as improvements that need to be made to your sleep pattern.

Going back to the quiz, it would be fairer to say that

feeling irritable is possibly related to poor sleep, but that other possible explanations should also be considered.

8. Most adults sleep 7–8 hours at night

How much sleep does a person need? As I have said, this is probably the most commonly asked question I come across. Unfortunately, there is not just one answer. The amount of sleep we need varies depending on our age, and on what we are doing in our lives. It also varies from person to person. It is important for people to discover their own personal sleep needs, at a particular point in time. That is one of the reasons you are using a sleep diary right now.

However, it is in fact TRUE that the average adult sleep is around 7 to 8 hours. If we take all adults from, say, 20 to 80 years and work out the average amount of sleep they have, it will be in the 7- to 8-hour range. We might then say that most adults sleep about this amount because the greatest proportion of people lie close to the average. The problem with averages, though, is that not everyone is the same. The average height of a male in the UK may be around 178 cm (5ft 10ins) but not everyone is that height! Many people are close to an average, but people are also different from each other, without that being abnormal. The same is true for sleep.

9. There is really no such thing as 'deep sleep'

The term 'deep sleep' sounds very much like what the general public might say, rather than a scientific description. You might think, therefore, that there is no such thing as deep sleep. However, this is a term that is also used in the research literature on sleep and in the clinical literature on sleep disorders. Deep sleep refers to non-REM stage 3 sleep, which are characterised by slow-wave EEG patterns. That is, the EEG waves are of high amplitude and low frequency, and are synchronised. These are sometimes called delta waves.

The answer to this question, therefore, is FALSE. Deep sleep *does* exist, and it is characteristic of our sleep, particularly during the first part of the night. In later life, older adults have much less slow-wave sleep, and so their non-REM sleep contains higher proportions of the lighter stage 2 sleep. In this sense older adults do not sleep as deeply as younger adults.

We need to be careful not to think that deep sleep is the best sleep. All types of sleep are important, and we need light sleep and REM sleep just as much as deep sleep. In fact, deep sleep accounts for a relatively small proportion of our total sleep (see Part One).

10. Daytime tiredness may be an important sign of a sleep disorder

I put this one in to help you consider the differences between tiredness and sleepiness. This is an important distinction to make. Tiredness is almost always present when people feel sleepy, but sleepiness is not always present when people feel tired. I think it is TRUE to say that daytime tiredness may be an important sign of a sleep disorder, but it is important to consider the extent to which you would also be at risk of falling asleep either when given the opportunity, or involuntarily.

There are a number of disorders which involve symptoms of excessive sleepiness, such as narcolepsy and sleep-related breathing disorder. Such disorders will not respond to CBT for insomnia, so it is important to identify them. One way to do this is to consider the tiredness–sleepiness dimension. People with insomnia commonly report feeling tired but do not necessarily report feeling that they are going to fall asleep. Quite the opposite: they tend to have difficulty getting to sleep . . . even during the day! We can also become sleepy at times when we are not getting enough sleep opportunity, e.g. through pressure of work causing us to cut short our time in bed, or through shift patterns.

11. Sleep problems usually pass away quite quickly

Of course, occasional sleep disturbance is very common. Everyone experiences difficulty getting to sleep or staying asleep at some time in their lives. It is TRUE that these problems usually sort themselves out and end up being short-lived. However, about 10 per cent of adults, that is one in ten people, experience persistent sleep problems, and this can be as high as one in five (20 per cent) in people over 65 years of age. There are probably even more people out there who suffer with insomnia but who do not seek help for it.

Sleep problems sometimes come in episodes, each time eventually passing but then recurring. When the pattern becomes one of persistent difficulty sleeping or repeated episodes that's a good time to seek help. Insomnia, once it has become established, can persist for many years. I guess that's why you are reading this?!

12. Most people don't cope very well after a bad night's sleep

Many people with sleep problems worry about them. They may worry about how they will cope, about having to take sleeping pills, about whether the insomnia is causing them serious harm and about whether it will ever go away. Although insomnia is distressing, and can be depressing, people often come to incorrect conclusions about their ability to sleep and the effects that sleeplessness will have.

Thoughts that run through our heads can make the problem much worse! Thinking 'I'm never going to get to sleep tonight' or 'I'll be hopeless at all the things I've got to do tomorrow' is *exaggerated* and is likely to get us more upset and make sleep even harder to come. Most people actually do manage to cope during the daytime even after a bad night's sleep – and you always get at least some sleep. In fact, only a proportion of people with insomnia feel tired after a bad night. You see – the body is designed to handle a certain amount of sleeplessness. It can be reassuring to know that even after a lot of lost sleep, it is not necessary to make it all up on other nights.

So, I have put this one down as FALSE because the question referred to 'most people' and for the majority the bad night doesn't become the norm. Of course, insomnia can cause problems with concentration, and we can feel tired, edgy and irritable. But we must remember to try to keep our thinking about sleep in proportion. After all, good sleepers get bad-tempered, too! The less you focus your concerns on sleep, the more you will succeed with sleep. If the question had been about *coping after a lengthy spell of bad sleep*, the answer would be rather different. As we have seen, chronic insomnia makes us vulnerable to developing depression and other mental health problems.

13. Sleeping pills are addictive

Although it may seem surprising, sleeping pills can affect our sleep in a negative way. The pills may help at first, but they often end up giving us problems rather than solving them, once our bodies become more and more used to them. Another thing is that many types of sleeping pills actually change the type of sleep we get, and they are not as good for us as a natural sleep. Because stopping some sleeping pills too quickly can cause severe insomnia, some people find that it is difficult to stop taking them. It is certainly TRUE, then, that some sleeping pills are dependency-forming, both physically and psychologically. You should bear in mind that any type of medication can become a behavioural habit just because we get used to taking them. I realise that 'addictive' is a strong word and you will see that I have spoken more about dependence, but at least this will get you thinking about the habits that we can get ourselves into if we rely on pills to sleep at night.

14. Taking a nap should be avoided if at all possible

If you absolutely have to take a nap because you are sleepy, then you should not try to prevent yourself from having that sleep. Resisting sleepiness can be dangerous. If you are sleepy rather than tired and fatigued, then I would be wondering why you feel so sleepy. Sleepiness is more associated with other types of sleep disorder than it is with insomnia, or it results from becoming sleep deprived.

So, this also is a difficult question to answer. If we take it from the perspective that you have insomnia, then I would say the answer to the question is TRUE. You should avoid taking a nap if it is at all possible, because napping during the day will reduce your homeostatic drive for sleep at night. A nap of more than around 10 minutes is likely to have some consequence for your ability to sleep at night, whereas short naps have a lesser impact, because they do not reduce the night-time sleep drive to the same extent.

15. Life changes can trigger insomnia

Everyone experiences stresses and strains in their day-to-day lives at home and at work, and there are times when these stresses can be severe. Such times can produce short-term sleep disturbance. However, temporary sleep problems do not always disappear even when problems have passed. This usually happens because our sleep schedule has been upset and poor sleep habits develop, or because we have learned to worry about not sleeping.

Changes in our lives, even positive changes like moving to a new house or switching to a better job, can also affect our sleep pattern. *Any* change is potentially stressful because we have to adapt to it. Some sleep difficulties are initially caused by health problems. Pain, discomfort or illness may upset us both physically and emotionally, and sleep problems may result. Similarly, psychological disorders like depression or anxiety can be associated with sleeplessness, but the insomnia can keep going even when we feel mentally stronger again. My conclusion, then, is that this is TRUE; life changes can trigger insomnia.

Did you identify any life events that might at first have triggered your sleep problem when you did your RAPIDLY formulation? Remember the 'A' stood for activate, and that was about triggers. Take a moment to look back at your notes and see what you wrote down. Jot down anything else that comes to mind now.

16. Some people seem to be able to do without sleep

I do not know of anyone who has ever been able to do without sleep, so this statement must be FALSE. In a manner of speaking, it may seem that some people hardly need any sleep, but the reality is that everyone does need sleep. Most people can manage to stay up for a night, or maybe two nights at a push, but that is a very short-term state of affairs and is definitely not advisable. Indeed, even if you do try to stay awake there is an increased chance of what we call microsleeps occurring without warning. This is where you have tiny sleep episodes for a few seconds. That's long enough to drive a car off the road when you come to a bend, and sadly accidents involving 'nodding off' happen all too often. If we allow a situation to develop where we are objectively sleepy and there is a risk that we are behaving dangerously it can end up as a criminal offence. Even the law of the land recognises that people cannot do without sleep.

17. Insomnia causes depression and depression causes insomnia

I am going to give the answer TRUE to this one. Insomnia and depression interact with each other, and in both directions.

Sleep disturbance is a common feature of a wide range of psychological and other mental disorders, including depression. Indeed, it is unusual to find someone with depression who does not have sleep disturbance. However, we also know from a large number of studies that insomnia symptoms often occur before depressive symptoms, and that having a persistent insomnia is a risk factor for the development of depression. So, it is just as accurate, to say that insomnia can cause depression.

There is a lot of research going on at the present time to help us figure out the exact relationship between insomnia and depression, as well as more generally about the role that sleep plays across the range of mental health problems. There is also the exciting prospect that overcoming insomnia might prevent or delay mental health problems developing. We know that treating depression on its own may not necessarily get rid of insomnia symptoms. So even if you are depressed, it would be useful for you to work through this CBT programme for insomnia alongside getting treatment for your depression.

18. I'd be better just giving up because I've tried it all before

To be honest, I put this statement in deliberately to be provocative. The answer, of course, is FALSE. You would be better learning more about how to overcome your insomnia!

Well, that's the quiz and those were my answers. How did you do? No harm in looking back over Part One if you want to brush up further on your sleep knowledge.

14

Putting Your CBT Programme Together

Introduction

Well, I have covered most of the CBT materials now.

I have encouraged you to assess your sleep problems, to formulate them using the RAPIDLY tool, and to navigate your personal journey through the cognitive, behavioural and relaxation therapeutic areas. Of course, I don't know whether you took the cognitive, behavioural or relaxation route first, and I don't know what you did next. I also don't know which particular techniques within each of these areas you chose to focus on. However, what I do know is that everything I have shared with you is known to be effective, so I'm confident that you are on your way to overcoming insomnia.

In this final chapter of Part Three, I want to reassure you that you can combine the techniques you have been learning. I'm sure that you have already been doing that, but I thought it would be valuable to devote some time to helping you put things together and to keep things altogether! The purpose of this chapter therefore is to help you integrate therapeutic elements from the programme and to help you to keep going until you have overcome your insomnia.

An overview of the CBT programme

In Box 22 I have summarised everything I have been saying to you about CBT and the support areas of sleep knowledge and sleep hygiene. I have structured it so that you can think of what to do in three important segments: before you got to bed, at bedtime, and if you can't sleep or if you wake up. I have also put in a few basics for consideration even before you start.

Now I do not expect that you will be using, or that you will need to use, every one of the twenty-five components that I have listed! My point is that the CBT ingredients can be put together to bake the CBT cake!

BOX 22: OVERVIEW OF THE CBT PROGRAMME

Some basics

1. Think of insomnia as a bad habit that can be corrected and stick to the programme until you establish a good habit.

2. Make sure you understand the idea of sleep efficiency – the proportion of the time you spend asleep when you are in your bed.

---

3. Work out your sleep schedule, your average sleep length, your planned rising time and threshold time for considering going to bed. Threshold time can be calculated by subtracting the average duration of your sleep at present from your planned rising time.

4. Make adjustments to your schedule at a maximum rate of 15 minutes per week and only after your sleep efficiency, the proportion of time spent asleep when in bed, reaches 90 per cent.

5. Always follow your planned sleep schedule 7 nights a week.

6. Practise your relaxation and imagery exercises until you have learnt them.

7. If you are considering reducing any sleeping pills that you take, consult your physician first to agree a plan, and reduce them gradually.

8. Use a sleep diary to record and track your progress.

9. Get a comfortable bed and mattress suitable to your needs and preferences.

10. Most importantly, get comfortable with CBT being challenging but definitely worth the effort!

Before you go to bed

11. Take light exercise in the late afternoon or early evening.

12. Put the day to rest long before bedtime. Think it through, tie up 'loose ends' in your mind and plan ahead. A notebook and diary will help to record and plan.

13. Wind down during the evening. Do not do anything mentally challenging within 90 minutes of bedtime, and stick to a routine.

14. Do not sleep or nap in the armchair. Keep sleep for bedtime.

15. Do not drink too much coffee or tea; eat a light snack for dinner and avoid eating chocolate and other products containing caffeine. Try to get used to de-caffeinated drinks.

16. Cut down your smoking in the evening and try not to smoke if you wake during the night.

17. Do not drink alcohol to aid your sleep – it usually upsets sleep.

18. Make sure your bed and bedroom are comfortable – not too cold, warm, noisy or bright. The room should be well aired and the alarm clock turned towards the wall.

19. Make preparations for waking during the night, such as leaving the heating on low in the living room and making a flask of a warm decaffeinated drink.

At bedtime

20. Stay out of bed until your threshold time and until you feel 'sleepy tired' – a tiredness that will make you fall asleep quickly and take you through the night.

21. Once in bed switch the light off immediately.

22. Do not read, watch TV, speak on the telephone, eat, drink, etc. in bed. The bedroom is for sleeping only, with the exception of sexual activity.

23. Practise relaxation exercises, followed by your imagery story. These procedures should be practised in the daytime before you try to apply them at night.

24. Give up trying to sleep. Keep your eyes open and gently resist sleep, or adopt a carefree or accepting attitude to wakefulness.

25. Remind yourself that sleep will come naturally. Repeat steps 23 and 24 as required.

26. Have your alarm set for the same rising time every day, 7 days a week, and make sure you rise at this time.

If you can't sleep or if you wake

27. If you can't sleep within quarter of an hour of putting the light out, get up and go into the living room.

28. Use the same rule above if you wake during the night and can't get back to sleep quickly.

29. Do something relaxing (planned beforehand) for a while when out of bed and do not worry about tomorrow.

30. Remind yourself that sleep problems are common and that you are working to overcome them. Try to avoid getting upset or frustrated.

31. Challenge all other intrusive and inaccurate ideas and mental images. Evaluate them and try to prevent them from dominating your thoughts.

32. Go back to bed when you feel 'sleepy tired' again. Put the light out and relax.

33. Try to block out unwanted thoughts by repeating the word 'the' to yourself every 2 seconds. Try to keep this up for 5 minutes at a time.

34. Write down any intrusive thoughts or concerns in a notebook kept at your bedside and deal with them in the morning.

35. If you still can't sleep then get up again after a quarter of an hour and repeat from step 27 onwards.

Why don't you note down or place a check mark (✔) against the techniques that you are using already and perhaps also mark (?) against those that you are thinking of as possible to add into the mix? Another tip would be look at the ones that you have neither ticked nor considered as possible. Think that through. Why have you excluded that one? Is it not relevant? Is it not possible? Don't misunderstand me, I am not suggesting that you do everything, but I do want to make sure that you are being thoughtful.

Developing a confident approach

A good sleep pattern may take quite a number of weeks to establish. You must be prepared for this. It is important, therefore, that you recognise the progress you are making along the way! There are two ways of measuring progress. First, are you getting better at implementing your therapy? If so, you are definitely making progress! Second, is your sleep pattern improving? You won't get the second without the first, so let's start with the implementation part!

Your progress in putting CBT into practice

Use the first column in Table 16 to write down what you have achieved so far. The simplest way would be to note down the item numbers from each of the sections in Box 22 that you are now managing to put into practice. Put the date at the top of the sheet, so you know where you stand right now. You can fill it in again in a couple of weeks and make a comparison, so you might want to make a copy of Table 16 or put the information in a notebook instead. Another alternative would be that you make up your own spreadsheet to record progress.

Table 16: Putting your CBT programme into practice

Progress Record   Date:

CBT components I am ACHIEVING	CBT components I am NOT ACHIEVING	CBT components I am NOT ACHIEVING	CBT components NOT RELEVANT TO ME

I know from experience that it won't be all good news! So, write down the item numbers that are still not achieved (or not fully achieved) in the second column. Everyone finds some parts of the programme more difficult than others. Don't be too discouraged by that. Instead, let's consider the reasons why.

One possibility is that some of the advice may not be particularly relevant for you. If that is the case, then you can shift that item number into the third column. For example, maybe you never did drink coffee, or don't have naps in the daytime anyway. Perhaps you don't have any problem falling asleep, so some of the things to do at bedtime don't seem necessary. If this is the kind of reason, then it won't matter too much. But just be sure you are not cheating with the items you are putting into column three!

Another possibility is that you can't quite get a grip of some part of what you are meant to be doing. My advice here would be to go back and re-read the relevant sections of the book and discuss anything you are confused about with someone you trust. I hope that this will clarify any points for you.

A third reason may be simply that what you are being asked to do is hard! It may be hard to remember a part of the programme because of old habits that are difficult to break, or it may be hard to motivate yourself to do something, or to stick at it. For example, it is not easy to get up out of bed if you don't fall asleep within a quarter of an hour, or to rise at the same time seven days a week. It can be very hard to change our behaviour. Likewise, we have to be quite strong in our minds to challenge negative and pessimistic thoughts so that they become more accurate and more encouraging . . . and it is not easy to give up trying to sleep!

You may feel a bit disheartened by the middle column where you have written down the list of items that you are a bit stuck with right now. All I can say is that I would be astonished if you were already managing to put all your therapy into practice all of the time! So, well done for all that you are doing. Try to be encouraged more than discouraged. Be firm but fair with yourself for what you have achieved. Nevertheless, you have an agenda there to work on. Why don't you set some goals for implementing the tricky bits, and write your goals down?

Your progress on your sleep measures

So, I hope your confidence is building now that you have a programme for overcoming your insomnia. I hope your confidence is growing, too, because your sleep has shown some improvement. Now would be a good time to re-visit the goals you wrote down at the start for what you were wanting to achieve. Are you getting closer to your goals?

Now is also a good time to measure your progress. Have you been sticking at using your sleep diary? It isn't absolutely essential, but I would strongly advice that you use it. You can also repeat your assessment on the sleep condition indicator from time to time.

Table 17: Evaluating progress using your sleep diary

Sleep Diary measure	Before CBT Date	Now Date	Follow-up Date	Follow-up Date	Follow-up Date	Follow-up Date
Wake-up time						
Rising time						
Bedtime						
Lights out						
Time in bed (lights out to rising time; mins)						
Time to fall asleep (mins)						
Number of wakenings						

Time awake during wakenings *(mins)*	Total time slept *(mins)*	Sleep efficiency *(Total time slept/Time in bed × 100)*	Sleeping pills *(number or mg)*	Alcohol *(units)*	Feeling rested after sleep *0, 1, 2, 3 or 4*	Sleep quality rating *0, 1, 2, 3 or 4*

I thought it might help if you had a table to summarise some of your sleep diary measures and how they have been changing over time. Have a look at Table 17.

The first column is for your sleep as it was at the start. You can transfer that information from your very first sleep diary. Just calculate some average scores for each item. The second column is for how your sleep is now; that is from your most recent diary. There are other columns that you can use in the future. In our research studies we do follow-ups at 1, 3, and 6 months, after completion of CBT programmes. By completing Table 17 you should be able to see the relationship between what you are doing in implementing the CBT programme (Table 16) and your progress with your sleep. Conducting this careful analysis of your sleep pattern and sleep quality will also help you see exactly where there has been some positive change, and exactly where there is still room for improvement.

I would encourage you to use your notebook to write down some maintenance goals and some improvement goals. Maintenance goals are your plans for keeping going with progress that has already taken place. For example, you might be falling asleep much more quickly now, so you want to make sure that you keep doing so! Your improvement goals would then be aspects of your sleep that still have some way to go. With the improvement goals, try to figure out how you can use the CBT programme to help yourself. Write down the conclusions you arrive at and the decisions you make about what to do. It may be that your record of putting CBT into practice (Table 16) will suggest things that need some extra work.

Trusting the evidence

Developing a confident approach is also about trusting the evidence. You are now gathering your own personal evidence about CBT for insomnia, but I just want to remind you that there is a lot of scientific evidence indicating that CBT is likely to work for you. We know from our studies that people keep on improving for at least 6 months after starting programmes like this. In many of our studies we have found continued improvement even a year later. Every encouragement then to keep on going! You will get more and more used to the changes that you have made, and you will reap more benefits. You have done the hard part so don't give up now.

Making lasting changes

Remember we are in this for the long game. I want to help you achieve change that will last.

We have been concentrating on examining changes that may be seen in your sleep pattern itself, but I hope there will be more than this for you. People I see at my Sleep Clinics often report benefits to their general well-being, not just to their sleep. This is because sleeping well is healthy and brings with it important bonuses. Improvements in energy levels, concentration, productivity, mood, general health and wellness, and quality of life are certainly possible over a period of months. In my experience these form part of the changes that can last. Have a think about whether you are beginning to see any generalised benefits like these just now, and write these down for your encouragement.

You will encounter obstacles on the way, be sure of that. In my line of work, we sometimes talk about something called relapse-prevention. Remember the wheel of motivation (Figure 17)? It tells us that we should expect at times to slip, so it is best to be prepared for that. Sometime or other you will get some bad nights and you will worry that you are in danger of being back at 'square one'. Relapse-prevention tells you first to expect that to happen, and second to reinstate all the elements of the CBT programme as soon as you can. If you feel that you are already doing these things and you can't understand why your sleep is disturbed, simply hold to your CBT programme, ride the storm, and it will probably rectify itself. Remember that acute sleep disturbance is essentially normal and temporary. It will tend to right itself as long as you don't get preoccupied with it.

You can also use this book as a form of booster therapy. This is a term we use in practice to describe how it often helps to give our progress a boost from time to time by refreshing on therapy. Just because you have read right through now doesn't mean that you have necessarily got the full benefit. Re-reading helps. Come back to the book to give yourself booster sessions on a regular basis. Why not even note some dates down right now as a future commitment to carrying on with the CBT approach?

Finally, keep in mind that your sleep efficiency and your sleep condition indicator scores are useful checks on how healthy your sleep is. I would encourage you to check your sleep condition every so often and also to estimate your sleep efficiency from time to time. You can make adjustments to your sleep window, as you have learned to do, and I am sure you will find that your sleep pattern becomes more regular and more satisfying. Given time you will find that you will be able to sleep without consciously using CBT techniques or methods.

Becoming a good sleeper

It must be a difficult thing to be a good sleeper, or so you would think! All this wind-down routine, relaxation and imagery, managing your arousal and your racing mind, establishing a strong bed–sleep connection, and getting your sleep pattern into shape. It all sounds pretty exhausting; like spinning lots of plates!

How on earth do good sleepers do it? How do they fit all this in? Good sleepers must be great jugglers! But then there is a special secret. Good sleepers are good sleepers precisely because what they do is second nature to them. As we have discovered, they just *don't* really think about it. Maybe they are not even the best at following good routines, and they do of course have some nights when they don't sleep well. My point is that the good sleeper is different from you because whatever they do is not done deliberately or anxiously to influence sleep. They are not preoccupied about sleep and so they sleep. And if they don't sleep so well . . . because they are not preoccupied about sleep, they tend not to get too concerned about it, so it sorts itself out. Remember the analogy of the dove?

In my experience the good sleeper is no student of sleep. Their sleep-related behaviour, the attitudes they have about sleep, and how they feel about sleep and about themselves as sleepers, simply supports sleep coming automatically and naturally. Nothing more, nothing less. 'So laid back as to be just about horizontal' is how the saying goes to describe someone who has a carefree approach. When it comes to sleep and the good sleeper, the saying, almost literally, has a ring of truth about it.

I want to help you to overcome insomnia *and* to become a good sleeper. For a while you have had to become a student of sleep, but to become a good sleeper in the end you must learn to mix the mind-set of the good sleeper into the CBT approach that you have been learning and applying. Although it may be hard to believe you will be able to sort things out and then forget about it, student days will be behind you!

Here's the final challenge. I need you for a while to stay 100 per cent committed to putting into practice all of the personalised programme I have given you. On the other hand, I need you to stop trying so hard and trust your sleep! Motivation and commitment to the programme are good; frantic effort and preoccupation are bad. I know from decades of experience that a steady, calm, and confident CBT approach is going to be effective for you.

My very best wishes to you in overcoming your insomnia, and in becoming a good sleeper!

PART FOUR

SPECIAL
CIRCUMSTANCES

Introduction to Part Four

The final part of this book comprises two brief chapters. They are relevant to you in the 'special circumstances' where you may need to consider what to do either about sleep medication, or about the possibility that you have a sleep disorder other than insomnia. Chapter 15 is about sleeping pills and Chapter 16 is about what we call 'differential diagnosis'.

15

What About
Sleeping Pills?

Introduction

Although this book is about CBT, I thought it would be
useful to include a brief chapter on sleeping pills. If you
are taking medication for your insomnia or are taking
some other kind of medicine that affects your sleep, you
must obtain advice from your prescribing physician. I want
to stress this point for two reasons. First, your physician
knows your overall physical and mental health and is best
qualified to give advice about your medicine management. Second, the comments that I have to make here can
only be taken as general in nature. They are *not* tailored
to meet your particular individual needs. This chapter,
therefore, should not be seen as an alternative to medical
consultation.

The broad purpose of this chapter is *to assist you in considering what place sleeping pills have in your sleep management plan.*
I hope what I have to say is useful to you.

327

The evidence about sleeping pills

Perhaps you have picked up this book because it is about CBT – which is a non-drug, or non-pharmacological approach to therapy. It may be that you are hoping to manage your sleep without using medication. Perhaps you prefer a non-drug approach to your health wherever that is possible. Perhaps you have been taking medication, but you are wondering about CBT instead.

Certainly, we live in an increasingly 'self-help' culture. If that means that people are becoming more and more interested in taking responsibility for their health, and for finding solutions to their health problems, then I think that must be a very good thing! Indeed, I wrote this book because I wanted to make what I know to be an effective treatment – CBT – directly available to people.

However, I am not in any fundamental sense against medication. Rather, my standpoint is that there is much stronger scientific evidence for the effectiveness of CBT than there is for sleeping pills when it comes to treating insomnia. CBT is what we call the *clinical guideline treatment of first choice* for persistent insomnia. This means that CBT is what clinicians are advised to recommend to their patients for an insomnia problem that has become *chronic*. That is *a difficulty getting to sleep and/or difficulty staying asleep that has been a problem three or more nights per week, for 3 months or longer, and is affecting the person's ability to function during the day.* By comparison there is much less evidence to support the use of sleeping pills, which are also known as *hypnotic drugs*, for persistent insomnia. So, the clinical guidelines suggest that medication should be the *second choice* treatment and only used if CBT is not effective on its own. To me, this is a matter of *evidence-based clinical practice* and not a matter of principle or philosophy.

The scientific *gold standard* is the *randomised controlled trial* (RCT). I have spoken about this before. When results of a number of RCTs are combined, something called a *meta-analysis* is produced (meta = many). RCTs and meta-analyses basically tell us what works most effectively, and advisory bodies use such studies as the evidence base on which they issue their guides to clinical practice. All the reviews of the evidence concerning sleeping pills come to the same conclusion: that sleeping pills are not recommended for persistent insomnia problems.

You will notice that I have been stressing persistent or chronic insomnia. This is because most people looking for help with their sleep have been having the problem for quite some time. In situations where the insomnia is more *short-term*, or what we call *acute*, medication may be more appropriate. Clinical guidelines suggest that taking a sleeping pill for a few nights, or very occasionally, can be helpful to improve sleep over the short term. As far as I am aware, there are no guidelines anywhere in the world, that recommend taking sleeping pills for months or for years under any circumstances.

I would rather not, but . . .

You may come to the matter of sleeping pills from the perspective that you would really rather not take them, but that you have found that they have given you at least some relief from insomnia. Perhaps it is difficult not to take them, especially in the absence of any real alternative. This is a huge problem. How can doctors and healthcare professionals advise CBT as the first-choice treatment if it isn't readily available?

I know this is why many people are using sleeping pills. Clinicians want to help their patients, but pills are often all that is available for the very large number of people who are looking for help with insomnia. We have spoken about *sleep hygiene*, but as you now know these lifestyle and bedroom changes are not sufficient to treat a chronic insomnia problem. Hopefully, this book on CBT will fill an important gap for you and for many others.

I have to acknowledge that it would be so much simpler if there was a sleeping pill that did the trick. CBT for insomnia involves quite a lot of hard work on your part . . . and it has taken me all of these pages to explain it to you! If the only instruction required was 'take this pill 30 minutes before bedtime', matters would be greatly simplified, and much less demanding for all concerned! Who knows, maybe in the future there will be a sleeping pill that guarantees restful good quality sleep for people with persistent insomnia. However, I do not see any such drug on the horizon at present.

A more likely development that will help solve the world-wide availability problem is CBT in digital form (dCBT). That is, CBT for insomnia delivered on web and mobile devices. I have been working on a dCBT programme called Sleepio™ over the past 10–15 years. We have conducted many large RCTs and these have been referenced in the clinical guidelines as showing an evidence base for this new dCBT approach. Sleepio™ is now available for some individuals in the United States and the United Kingdom as a covered benefit or as part of their healthcare. I will provide more information on this in the section headed 'useful organisations'.

Do I need to stop?

I think a lot of people go to their general practitioner worried that, one of these days, the doctor is going to refuse to prescribe any more sleeping pills. Certainly, I can think of patients who have felt that they were in the 'last chance saloon'! They may have been told that they can have pills for one more week or one more prescription, or have been advised to 'make them last'. Patients commonly recognise that they have gone the full circle with medication and have not found anything that really solves the problem. Yet, the prospect of stopping may be very daunting.

Physicians are under quite a bit of pressure not to prescribe treatments unless they are known to be effective, or unless they are clearly benefiting the individual patient. This can lead to quite a bit of momentum from the physicians' side to encourage you to stop or to severely limit what you take.

Of course, stopping is important to patients too . . . and may well be part of your goal in following this CBT programme. Indeed, often patients say to me that they would feel much better about themselves if they could get off their medication. It is like a goal in its own right to sleep naturally again. So, what is the answer to the question 'do I need to stop?'

My advice to you would be to 'take the bull by the horns'. Go along to your prescribing physician and have an honest discussion about your use of sleep medications. Discuss the specific medication that you are taking and the length of time you have been on it. Discuss the potential benefits of staying on the pills relative to the benefits, and the difficulties, in stopping or *withdrawing*. Discuss whether or not there are any other pharmacological options. I am sure you would have your physician's respect for doing this. I think decisions about medication should always be a *partnership* between the patient and the physician. Ask your physician if you can agree a joint plan, based upon what would be best for your health. That plan might well be a reduction schedule. You should also explain that you are following my structured CBT programme, and describe a bit about the content of the programme.

Off-label prescribing for chronic insomnia

The lack of availability of CBT, coupled with the absence of a safe and effective sleeping pill for chronic insomnia has led to a great deal of what is called *off-label prescribing* for insomnia. That is where medicines that are not officially approved for insomnia are prescribed instead of the approved sleeping pill medicines. Please don't misunderstand what I'm saying. These off-label drugs are approved drugs, but their approvals are for other conditions, not for insomnia. This is what the off-label term means.

Doctors are not doing anything wrong in prescribing them, it's just that they are prescribing these off-label drugs for a condition (in this case insomnia) for which they are not intended. Most commonly, these are drugs that cause sleepiness as a side-effect. A good example would be what is known as a *tricyclic or sedative anti-depressant* drug. These are meant, as you can see, to treat depression but because they also make people drowsy, they are quite commonly offered in a low dose to people with insomnia, even when the person is not depressed.

As I say, discuss your medication regime with your physician. I have summarised the main types of drugs that are used for insomnia in Table 18.

Can I take sleeping pills and use CBT?

Again, this is a question that my patients raise. So, we should also consider the possibility that there may be some benefit associated with taking sleep medication as well as following the CBT programme. This too is something you could discuss with your physician.

After all, if medication affords some short-term benefit to sleep, and CBT is effective in the long-term, would it not be possible to capitalise on a combined sleeping pill plus

CBT approach? In many ways this is an attractive idea. It is also a very important research question, because in practice this combination is quite common. There are some data to suggest a combination can work, but the combination doesn't work any better than CBT on its own.

As far as I can see from my reading there is no clear advantage for planning to combine CBT with sleeping pills, except possibly in the first few weeks. If someone is already taking medication, then of course adding CBT may be a good step. Likewise, if someone is not responding enough to CBT alone then adding medication is recommended as an option in the clinical guidelines.

However, there are also a couple of potential problems to look out for. One is that taking sleeping pills may reduce your attention to the CBT programme, because taking pills is relatively easy by comparison! Another is that problems of *attribution* can arise with combination therapies. This is because you can never be sure what is causing any benefit that you experience. For example, you could (incorrectly) attribute treatment effects to the medication and so slacken off or even abandon some of the CBT methods. This would be likely to lead to a poor outcome because, of the two, CBT is the proven treatment. It could also lead in extreme cases to the development of dependency on medication.

How can I come off pills safely?

If you have decided that you want to stop taking sleeping pills, then you must consult your physician. However, I can provide you with some general guidelines on good practice for safe withdrawal. Please bear in mind that I am referring here to sleeping pills not to off-label prescriptions which are different types of drugs and will have different chemical properties.

Over a period of time in taking sleeping pill medication, your body becomes used to the drug's chemistry and to the concentration levels of the drug in your bloodstream. This process is known as *tolerance*. It is because of the build-up of tolerance that you may have experienced that the drug doesn't work as well as it used to work, or you have had to take a higher dose of your sleep medication in order to get the same effect. The fact that your body may have become used to the medication is one reason why a *gradual reduction* in medication is essential.

Of course, the concentration of a drug in your bloodstream is something that is constantly changing as your body metabolises or breaks down the chemical components of the drug. Different drugs are metabolised at different rates, and to give an indication of the length of time it takes our bodies to clear a compound, we use the term *half-life*. Half-life is the time (in hours) it takes for components of the drug to reduce their concentration by 50 per cent. I do not know which particular pills you have been taking, so I can only give you general advice, and of course encourage you to speak to your doctor.

So called 'short-acting' drugs reach their peak concentrations in the bloodstream quickly and are eliminated quickly, whereas 'long-acting' drugs are usually slower to act, but also take much longer to clear. The advantage of short-acting

Table 18: Medications sometimes used for insomnia. Some drugs are not available in certain territories. Those marked * are off-label

Family of drug	Examples of drugs	Comments
Benzodiazepine receptor-acting	Nitrazepam, Flurazepam, Loprazolam, Lormetazepam, Temazepam, Triazolam	These are the traditional sleeping pills.
	Zaleplon, Zolpidem, Zopiclone, Eszopiclone	The last four ('z' drugs) are more recent.
Orexin receptor antagonists	Suvorexant	These are newer sleeping pills with a different mechanism of action to the class above.
	Lemborexant	
Melatonin receptor agonists	Ramelteon	These are clinical grade drugs that promote melatonin.
	Agomelatine	
	Circadin	

WHAT ABOUT SLEEPING PILLS?

★ Antidepressants	Trimipramine Doxepin Trazodone	These are drugs licensed for depression. Trimipramine and doxepin are tricyclic antidepressants.
★ Dopamine serotonin antagonists/neuroleptics	Quetiapine Olanzepine Risperidone Clozapine	These are drugs typically used for psychosis. They used to be called major tranquilisers.
Over-the-counter/health products	Diphenhydramine (antihistamine), L-tryptophan (amino acid), valerian (herb), melatonin (hormone)	These are non-prescription products with no clinical efficacy for insomnia.

sleeping pills is that, being more rapidly being eliminated from the body chemistry, they tend to have fewer *carry-over effects* into the next day. By comparison long-acting sleeping pills can lead to carry-over morning drowsiness. Although short-acting drugs avoid this particular problem, they are on the other hand more prone to *withdrawal effects*, because of their rapid elimination from the blood chemistry. Longer acting drugs withdraw more slowly and have a less abrupt withdrawal profile.

As you will see in Table 18, I have listed the main classes of drugs that are commonly prescribed by doctors to promote sleep. Only those in the top half of the table are licensed as sleeping pills. I have identified medications that are used in off-label prescribing; and also noted over-the-counter (OTC; non-prescription) remedies. These OTC products offer no known clinical benefits to insomnia.

No doubt you will have heard people talking about having a 'fast metabolism' or a 'slow metabolism'. This reflects another important consideration. Medication should be prescribed and withdrawn *on an individual basis*. As a general rule, for example, older adults metabolise drugs more slowly and eliminate them more slowly, which means that older adults on certain medications are more likely to experience carry-over effects.

So, I would stress that there is no absolute recommended withdrawal rate if you are planning to try to do without sleeping pills. You really need to consult your physician. What I have done though is to provide you in Table 19 with a few pointers concerning a sleeping pill reduction schedule. You will see that it is particularly important that any withdrawal process should follow a gradual *taper*.

Table 19: General advice on sleeping pill withdrawal

1. Always consult your doctor when you are considering reducing or stopping sleep medication.

2. Obtain advice on a planned withdrawal schedule that suits your individual requirements. A suitable plan may require weeks to complete.

3. Always reduce sleep medication by gradual tapering. Usually, small reductions in the medication dosage, or in the frequency of doses, will be advised by your doctor. Commonly reductions will be 25 to 50 per cent of the dosage, at intervals of one to two weeks.

4. Do not take additional medications or substitute medications unless they have been prescribed for you.

5. Tapering schedules should be reviewed weekly, or more frequently if you experience severe withdrawal effects.

6. Once you get down to the lowest prescribed dosage for each night, your doctor may recommend having 'drug holidays'. This is where you skip nights from taking this lowest dose, gradually skipping more and more nights until you stop altogether.

7. Keep a careful note (in your sleep diary and notebook) of your medication use, sleep pattern, and experiences associated with the withdrawal period.

8. Staying off sleeping pills can be difficult. Try to prevent relapse by identifying situations coming up that might tempt you to take medication, and use CBT instead.

Can CBT help me to come off sleep medication?

Sometimes people want to know if they can replace their sleep medication with CBT. They want to be able to trust another method and hope that CBT may provide them with that opportunity. I think that this is a realistic possibility, but you need to think through what is likely to be the most successful means to that end for you. There are basically three options. All this is assuming you are following a gradual taper under medical supervision.

The first option is to withdraw medication gradually before commencing CBT. I will call this the 'withdraw before' method. The main advantage here is that you can see what your underlying sleep pattern is like, before starting CBT. As long as you have finally come off your sleeping pills for a few weeks, the withdraw before option allows you to get a proper baseline on your sleep. It may even be that you won't require to start CBT if your sleep improves spontaneously once the medication is withdrawn. This does happen in some cases! The disadvantage, of course, is that it may not be easy to discontinue sleeping pills without some other strategy already in place.

The second option would be to 'withdraw after' CBT. The advantage here is that you don't need to start with the challenge of doing without pills and can concentrate straight away on the CBT programme. If you see that your sleep is improving, then you may gain sufficient confidence in CBT to enable you to withdraw after. The disadvantage though is that your sleep pattern is likely to get disrupted again once the withdrawal process begins, and this might be difficult to take if you have only recently begun to sleep better! You should not expect that using CBT will mean that you can bypass drug withdrawal effects, although it may help you cope with them better.

The third option is to 'withdraw during' CBT. This might feel like you are getting the best compromise of the advantages I have expressed above. However, you should bear in mind the disadvantage that it may be quite difficult to figure out how changes in your sleep pattern relate to the two things (CBT, withdrawal) that are going on at the same time.

How do you choose between them? Well, I don't actually consider that this question is as hard to answer as you might think! My advice would be to follow the option that you are most likely to be able to carry through in practice. In other words, be *pragmatic* about this! The most important thing is to be able to take advantage of what CBT can offer and to stop medication if you and your doctor feel it is not benefiting you.

16

Recognising and Managing Other Common Sleep Disorders

Introduction

At various points throughout the book I have mentioned the importance of checking that you *do* have insomnia . . . and checking that you *do not* have a different type of sleep problem. It is possible that you could have more than one sleep disorder, of course; we call this comorbidity. In which case it is worth getting that other disorder checked out, even though CBT may still help your insomnia.

In Part One, I introduced you to the sleep disorders and in Part Two, I gave you some tools to help you to assess your sleep pattern and sleep symptoms. Have a look back at the self-assessment you went through using Table 4. This was a sleep disorder 'screening' procedure. Let me now introduce another bit of jargon that we use in clinical practice!

Clinicians are trained in what is known as *differential diagnosis*. That is the skill of distinguishing one type of disorder from another type of disorder. When you are unwell you usually seek advice at first from a general medical practitioner, who begins the process of differential diagnosis. If it is thought that you need more specialised investigation or assessment, you may be referred on to someone else for an opinion. These days, diagnostic and treatment skills are becoming increasingly specialised, in every area of medicine. Sleep is no exception, and we now have clinicians who are sleep specialists; people with advanced training and certification in the field of *Sleep Medicine*. Often these physicians are Neurologists or Pulmonologists (respiratory specialists). The sub-specialty that specialises in insomnia management has become known as *Behavioural Sleep Medicine* and the majority of these professionals are Clinical Psychologists.

So, what can you possibly do for yourself?! It sounds quite complicated. Well, I am not suggesting that you should do your own differential diagnosis. There is some truth in the saying that a little knowledge can be a bad thing. On the other hand, I think it is very helpful for you to be well informed about the key symptoms of different types of sleep disorder, so that if you do need to consult a professional you can have a more informed discussion about things. In particular, your answers to questions in Table 4 should help raise your awareness about five different groups of sleep disorders that may need different approaches to management from insomnia. If you think that any of these might apply to you then you should make an appointment to see your physician.

The aim of this chapter, therefore, is to *assist you to consider the possibility that you may have a sleep disorder other than insomnia and to take steps to seek appropriate help.*

Table 20: Sleep disorders other than insomnia: summary of symptoms

Type of sleep disorder	Symptoms
Circadian disorder	*Delayed sleep phase syndrome* – awake till late, difficulty initiating sleep, difficulty waking in morning, still sleepy if rising at normal rising time, sleep normally if you go to bed very late and rise very late
	Advanced sleep phase syndrome – evening sleepiness, difficulty delaying sleep till normal bedtime, early morning wakening, sleep normally if you go to bed very early and rise very early
Sleep-related breathing disorder	*Obstructive sleep apnoea* – loud snoring (in most cases), breathing pauses, fragmented sleep with micro-arousals, daytime sleepiness, sometimes flat/ depressed, often overweight
Restless legs and limb movements in sleep	*Periodic limb movement disorder* – involuntary jerky movements interrupting sleep, repetitive pattern of movements, may have daytime sleepiness
	Restless legs syndrome – irresistible urge to move legs when at rest, causing arousals from sleep
Parasomnias	*Sleepwalking* – occurs during incomplete arousals from deep sleep (stage 3, slow wave sleep), difficult to waken, usually amnesic for event

	Night terrors – occurs during incomplete arousals (as in sleepwalking), often sit up in bed, strong emotional display, difficult to comfort or waken, usually amnesic for event
	Sleeptalking – normally occurs during transitions between sleep stages
	Confusional arousals – arise on emerging from non-REM sleep, strange and confused behaviour, may be hard to comfort
	Nightmares – emotionally laden dream content, often waken frightened from REM sleep
	Teeth-grinding (nocturnal bruxism) – occurs in different stages of sleep and at transitions
	REM behaviour disorder – muscle tone retained during REM sleep, dream enactment often aggressive
Narcolepsy and hypersomnia	Full narcolepsy syndrome comprises:
	Sleep attacks – sudden involuntary sleeps in the daytime
	Hypersomnia – excessive sleepiness and extended sleeps
	Cataplexy – sudden loss of muscle tone in major muscle groups, in response to emotion
	Hypnagogic/hypnopompic hallucinations – dream-like hallucinations upon entering/leaving sleep
	Sleep paralysis – inability to move voluntarily, especially when emerging from sleep

Disorders of the body clock (circadian disorders)

I am going to say a bit more about circadian disorders of sleep than about the other categories which follow because these disorders are more commonly confused with insomnia.

We learned earlier on that some body clock functions are age-related. For example, the sleep drive of young adults can remain strong at 7 in the morning, compared to older adults where it begins to decline from about 5 in the morning. Later life is also associated with increases in sleepiness in the middle part of the evening. Another factor may simply be individual differences. Some people, regardless of age, have always tended to be 'larks' and others have tended to be 'owls'. So, it is important that you consider both your age and your typical sleep time preferences before concluding that you have a circadian sleep disorder. In Table 20 there are two sub-categories of circadian problem that I want to mention. Let's take each of these in turn.

Delayed sleep phase syndrome (DSPS) often develops at a young age. You may not be surprised when you consider the key symptoms. This circadian disorder may present as a sleep-onset insomnia – that is difficulty initiating sleep. Central to the complaint is an inability to get to sleep at the desired time . . . but there is also an inability to wake up at the desired time. In other words, the person with DSPS is out of step with the world by falling asleep late and waking and rising late. You might say 'typical of a teenager', but for the person with DSPS this has not just been a temporary stage of growing up. Another feature is that there is usually little night-to-night variability in sleep pattern. The person with DSPS can, if left to their own 'out of phase' schedule, have a normal sleep of good quality. They will fall asleep quickly (late on), sleep right through ('sleep in'), and the EEG sleep stage distribution of their sleep will be normal. Typically, if they try to get up at a more normal hour (say 7 a.m.) they will remain drowsy for some hours until their body clock reaches its wake time.

Another reason why DSPS might develop, and it applies to other circadian problems for that matter, is when people have been *working shifts*, and then try to get back into an 11 p.m. to 7 a.m. sleep pattern. Usually, people begin to adjust after a couple of weeks, but there are those who find this much harder. *Jet lag* is an even more common experience that also is usually temporary. Typically, it takes anything from a few days or up to around 10 days for your body clock to adjust to a different time zone. The bigger the time difference the more adjustment there is of course. Nevertheless, it seems that people differ in their adaptability to these different types of circadian problem because adolescence, shift work and international travel affect some people much more than others!

Advanced sleep phase syndrome (ASPS) is really just the opposite of DSPS. In ASPS, problems are associated with early settling to sleep and with early morning wakening. It is hard to 'keep going' during the evening because sleepiness kicks in early, and it may well be impossible to sustain sleep beyond 3 a.m. or 4 a.m., or even earlier in extreme cases. ASPS is also the opposite of DSPS because it is more common in older people, rather than younger people. Furthermore, the fragmentation of sleep in later life may lead to daytime napping, and this can contribute further to an already compromised sleeping and waking routine.

I should point out of course that our lifestyles play a part in determining circadian disorders of the DSPS and ASPS variety. I have already mentioned the 'enforced' lifestyle of shift work and, of course, there is peer pressure for young people to stay up late. However, *lifestyle choices* may also be implicated in the development of sleep phase disorders. For example, retired people may choose to retire early to bed because their lifestyle does not necessitate staying up late for a whole variety of reasons. In sleep science we talk of *zeitgeber*s or 'time-givers'. These are the factors that determine the social rhythm of our lives – our routines if you like. Developmental, social and personal factors may all be zeitgebers. However, where sleep and wakefulness are concerned, natural light is really the chief zeitgeber of all! Generally speaking, we sleep when it is dark, and we are awake in the daylight. I covered this in Part One and explained about *melatonin*, the pineal hormone that plays a central part in regulating bodily rhythms.

So how would you know if you had circadian disorder rather than insomnia? Well, first of all consult the key symptom checklist in Table 20. Also go back over the relevant part of the sleep history I gave you in Table 3 and the screener in Table 4. Another thing you can do is to look through your sleep diaries. I suggest taking at least two consecutive weeks, and longer if you can. Do you find that you tend to go to bed early and to waken early? Do you sleep well if you allow yourself to follow that routine? If so, ASPS is worth considering. Do you find that you don't properly waken up until hours after you rise in the morning? Do you find that you never get to sleep until the 'small hours'? If so, then you could have DSPS.

If you can get access to an actigraphic assessment of your sleep this also helps with the diagnosis. An *actigraph* is a medical grade device that is much superior to the wearable devices that you can buy in the store or online. The actigraph is worn like a wristwatch and measures body movement and stores the information in an internal microchip for computer analysis. Active and inactive periods across several weeks are then displayed graphically, and it is possible to see what times of the day and night the natural peaks and troughs in movement occur. If they are out of alignment with the normal sleep (inactive) and wake (active) cycles, then this might suggest that you have a circadian problem. We are moving here into specialised assessment though. You can't expect to get this kind of work up at your local GP. So, I would suggest that if you suspect DSPS or ASPS, you should take this thought to your GP and discuss with your GP what to do next. There are several options that might be considered.

Sometimes just *re-scheduling* your sleep strictly, and gradually shifting your bedtime and rising time can be effective. The aim is to move steadily closer and closer to the normal bedtime hours. For example, let's suppose the problem is

DSPS and you think that you are 3 hours out of line (getting sleepy at 2 a.m. and remaining sleepy till around 10 a.m.). You might start by sleeping 2 a.m to 10 a.m. for one week, then shift to 1.45 a.m. to 9.45 a.m. in week two, then to 1.30 a.m. – 9.30 a.m. during week three, and so on, until you get to your desired schedule. If you had ASPS, you would re-schedule too, but in the opposite direction of course!

There is some evidence that one of the melatonin receptor agonist drugs (see Table 18) can improve sleep timing, so it may be useful for DSPS and ASPS. This is something you should discuss with your physician of course. There is also some evidence that *bright light therapy* can be used to improve circadian rhythm. This is connected to the melatonin story because, as we learned before, bright light shuts down the brain's production of melatonin. In DSPS, bright light in the morning can help to 'phase advance' the major sleep period, and in ASPS, bright light in the evening can help to phase delay sleep. Light boxes are commercially available in stores and on the web. If you want to use one of these, you should again take care to read instructions and limitations. The evidence seems to be that 10,000 *lux* for 30 minutes is about right to have a therapeutic effect.

It may be possible to combine the use of re-scheduling, melatonin and light therapy, and you can often also use CBT because sleep phase disorders and insomnia often occur together. As with the diagnosis of DSPS or ASPS, the treatment of circadian disorders should be conducted under skilled supervision. Certainly, consult your physician and consider the possibility of referral to a specialised sleep disorders clinic.

Sleep Related Breathing Disorders (SBD)

This term refers to a group of disorders that seriously disrupt the continuity of sleep through impaired breathing. In some countries this field is known as *respiratory* medicine, in others the term *pulmonary* medicine is used. Either way, the point is that when breathing is affected during sleep, the quality of sleep that a person gets is likely to be poorer.

The most obvious and common example that comes to mind is *snoring*. Many people snore. This does not mean that they necessarily have a clinical problem with their sleep. Snoring is simply the sound made by the passage of air across a restricted airway. During sleep there is a tendency for the airway to 'collapse' (get narrower) so there is more respiratory effort involved in drawing air through the nose. Of course, air contains the *oxygen* that sustains life, so as long as the brain can tell that we are getting enough oxygen into the bloodstream there is no problem – except perhaps for the partner having to listen to the noise!

However, if there is not enough air getting through, the bloodstream becomes *deoxygenated* or *desaturated*. These are just terms we use to describe the unsatisfactory situation where oxygen levels are below the level that is necessary to maintain good sleep. Fortunately, the brain 'reads' this situation and causes us to arouse from sleep towards wakefulness, so that more normal breathing can recommence.

It is possible for people who do not snore to have respiratory problems of this kind, so you should be aware of that. However, snoring, being overweight and having a thick-set neck (with a collar size of 17 inches or more) are all closely related to sleep-related breathing disorders.

There is increasing public awareness of an SBD known as *obstructive sleep apnoea* (OSA). In OSA, the upper airway collapses primarily during stages 1 and 2 of sleep; that is the lighter forms of non-REM sleep, as well as during REM sleep. An 'apnoea' is a complete closure/blockage of the upper airway. We call this an *occlusion* of the airway. Basically, breathing stops! Partial, or incomplete, occlusions may also occur, and these are known as 'hypopneas'. In OSA apnoeaic and hypopneaic events disrupt sleep by causing *micro-arousals*. These brief wakenings are enough to cause *sleep fragmentation* and less refreshing sleep.

How would you know if you might have an SBD like OSA? Well, your most obvious night-time symptoms would be very heavy snoring and difficulty remaining asleep. You might even be conscious of a tendency to waken out of sleep catching your breath, or of a feeling that you had stopped breathing. Some people waken themselves up with the sudden re-starting of their breathing after an apnoea. Also speak to your partner. Your partner may be aware of your breathing pattern, your snoring, and may have witnessed these 'breathing pauses'. Sometimes people with OSA waken with a headache and a very dry mouth in the morning.

OSA is associated also with daytime symptoms. The most important of these is *excessive daytime sleepiness*. Here there may be an involuntary tendency to fall asleep when at rest, or even when undertaking activities. Problems with concentration and irritability are often reported in OSA and sleepiness has been linked to an increased likelihood of road traffic and industrial accidents. This is not a disorder to be taken lightly because yourself and others can be at risk due to the daytime sleepiness symptom causing accidents. SBDs have also been associated with increased risk of medical disorders, particularly of the cardiovascular system.

Clinical diagnosis of an SBD can only be confirmed through specialised assessment. These PSG assessments include not only the standard sleep set-up (EEG, EOG, EMG) but also measurement of respiration and of blood-oxygen saturation levels (see Figure 1). Of course, assessment would also include a detailed interview, and partners are often invited to attend, for the reasons I mentioned above. If you suspect that you may have an SBD, you should consult your physician. Certainly, if you have daytime sleepiness problems there is a distinct possibility that your sleep at night needs some investigation. Your physician will know where to refer you.

Regarding treatment, *positional advice* to maximise breathing and to prevent airways collapse, and *weight loss* may be beneficial. Some dental *prosthetic devices* are also available. These are normally 'made to measure' and are worn in the mouth to improve breathing during sleep. Most of these devices serve to advance the lower jaw and extend the airway. *Surgery* is also used in some severe cases of OSA to rectify problems more permanently. At the symptomatic level, some *medications* stimulate arousal and reduce daytime sleepiness, but this is more controversial.

The mainstay of treatment for OSA, however, is known as *continuous positive airway pressure*. CPAP (for short) is a simply a mechanical pump, which delivers a steady stream of air during sleep. This air is delivered under sufficient pressure to support the upper airway and to prevent airway collapse. Unfortunately, CPAP is not an elegant treatment! The most common clinical practice is to recommend use of a special mask that fits over the nose and is held in place by headgear consisting of straps. The mask is connected to a flexible tube through which air is delivered from the pump machine that sits on the bedside table.

The good news though is that CPAP is very effective at eliminating breathing pauses. So, the natural pattern of sleep is restored, without interruption, and daytime symptoms reduce markedly. Normally people need to keep on using their CPAP machine long-term if they want to stay symptom free. Some people with OSA also have insomnia. If that is the case it is best to follow your CBT as well, but don't neglect to get sleep breathing problems evaluated if you are concerned about them.

Restless legs and limb movements in sleep

Periodic limb movement disorder (PLMD) *and restless legs syndrome* (RLS) are disorders that may occur in people who have SBD, or they may present in the absence of such breathing disorders. Again, there are no psychological treatments for PLMD or RLS and both conditions require careful assessment.

PLMD is mainly associated with older age, and involves muscle twitches in the limbs, particularly the legs, during sleep. These episodes of involuntary movement disrupt sleep, causing arousals mostly from light sleep, leading to complaints of daytime sleepiness and insomnia. The diagnosis of PLMD is generally confirmed by PSG. As well as the standard PSG set up that I described in Part One, for this type of sleep study electrodes are also attached to the major leg muscles to pick up any signs of jerky or restless leg movements that might be related to brief sleep arousals and sleep fragmentation (Figure 1).

Of course, most people have experienced the occasional involuntary limb movement. For example, many people get what we call *hypnic jerks* or *sleep starts* from time to time. These are sudden, brief jerky movements that occur at or around sleep-onset and waken us from light sleep. Hypnic jerks sometimes become a problem in their own right, but for most people they happen rarely. In some ways the movements in PLMD are similar to this except they occur repeatedly and throughout the night. We do not know exactly why people get PLMD. It may be related to disturbance of circadian sleep-wake rhythms in later life or to specific disorders of motor function that again occur more commonly in older adults. However, there are some medications that help PLMD. The options are either sedative type drugs of the benzodiazepine family that reduce muscle function during sleep, or 'dopaminergic' agents that are used to treat neuromuscular disorders.

RLS, as the name suggests, involves periods of irresistible urges to move the legs. These episodes are associated with unpleasant cramping sensations in the legs that are relieved only by walking or other movement or exercising of the legs. The symptoms begin mostly in the evening, potentially delaying the onset of sleep. So, they may occur when a person is resting or relaxing, and not only during sleep itself. When they interfere with sleep the usual result is sleep fragmentation and arousals. People with RLS may also suffer from significant daytime sleepiness. Normally people with RLS are able to give a clear picture of their problem and they may have had it a long time. Although many people with RLS are of middle age or older, about one-third of cases have their first symptoms before the age of 20 years.

The background to RLS is also a bit of a mystery, but like PLMD, there may be associated changes in dopamine neurotransmission. Some of these may be age-related. RLS has also been associated with pregnancy and with end-stage renal (kidney) disease. In pregnancy it usually presents in the third trimester and can be alleviated with iron supplementation, but typically resolves after the birth. Treatment of RLS is similar to that for PLMD, and indeed PLMD and RLS commonly occur together.

Sleepwalking, night terrors and other parasomnias

The *parasomnias* are a group of disorders that intrude into the sleep process and create disruptive behavioural events. They are associated with disorders of arousal, of partial arousal, or of transitions between different stages of sleep. Non-REM parasomnias are quite common during childhood and in most instances, they resolve quite naturally. That is, they just disappear. However, they can also persist into adulthood, or less commonly, present then for the first time. The most common presentations of non-REM parasomnia include *sleepwalking (somnambulism)*, *sleeptalking (somniloquy)*, *night terrors* (sometimes called *sleep terrors*), and disorientation or confusion upon wakening (*confusional arousals*). These disorders are often referred to as incomplete arousals out of deep sleep.

Other parasomnias include REM sleep disorders, such as *REM behaviour disorder* (RBD). This is characterised by an absence of the 'muscle atonia' that is normally present during REM sleep. In other words, someone with RBD may have retained motor function during dreaming sleep. So, the person with RBD may be able to act out their dreams, carrying out complex, and seemingly purposeful behaviour while remaining physiologically asleep. Consequently, such parasomnias and their associated behaviours – particularly sleepwalking and dream enactment, may lead to personal injury or injury to the bed partner. On rare occasions people have been known to carry out relatively complex tasks, like driving a car, or criminal acts including murder during a parasomnia episode.

Exactly when in the night a parasomnia event occurs is often crucial in determining the underlying sleep disorder. For example, night terrors occur in stage 3 non-REM sleep, often towards the end of the first or second phase of deep sleep. Therefore, like sleepwalking, they present more commonly during the first third of the night. Because incomplete arousals out of deep sleep are involved, people who sleepwalk or have night terrors rarely have any accurate recall of what they were doing or what was on their mind at the time. This may seem surprising to the observer because the sleepwalker may appear purposeful in their activity, perhaps even trying to get out of the house or to find something. Similarly, a night terror is very distressing to watch because the person experiencing it appears extremely emotional and in a state of high physiological arousal and agitation. It is because the arousal is not a complete one and because the stage of sleep is a deep one that there is no conscious memory trace. Even if you do waken a sleepwalker or rouse someone from a night terror, they tend to remain 'groggy' and have only fleeting images or emotional statements to report. Sometimes the problem evolves into what we call a *confusional arousal* and this can last for some time.

By contrast, *nightmares* occur during REM sleep, which is as we have learned, a relatively light form of sleep. They also relate more to the second half of the night, when REM episodes are more prolonged. These events often end with the dreamer actually waking up, so the memory trace is laid down more vividly. Indeed, because nightmares usually involve frightening or bizarre images or stories, arousal from sleep is not only abrupt but clear, and the person is unable to get back to sleep easily. We say in our jargon that the person with nightmares usually has *narrative recall* for the occurrence and content of these dream events. That is the storyline is retained; and sometimes it can be recurrent.

Having a better understanding of what is going on is the best treatment for all the parasomnias. *Information, education* and *reassurance* are very important. Indeed, I quite often find, once I have explained the symptoms and given the diagnosis, that patients with these problems don't need to come back to the clinic. We usually discover that there is an early history, of say being prone to sleepwalk, and that some current stress factor has brought about a recurrence. Sometimes though people haven't acknowledged that they are under a strain – so be warned! On occasions I say to people that their parasomnia is 'like a friend tapping them on the shoulder and asking if they are sure they are OK'. So, if you are the kind of person who copes with things very well on the surface, but you tend to bury things you don't like to face, or if you bottle them up – then you will know I am speaking to you!

Other things can make parasomnias more of a problem. *Sleep deprivation* is to be avoided because if you are not getting enough sleep, the homeostatic pressure for sleep builds up. Too many late nights, particularly when accompanied by a change in life circumstances, can be fertile ground for parasomnias to present on the 'recovery' nights. You see, in these circumstances your deep sleep and your REM sleep, two important sleep types, can go into 'rebound'. That is, your body prioritises them as it tries to catch up on lost sleep. Consequently, the likelihood of parasomnia increases because you spend more time in the sleep states that 'host' parasomnia problems.

A related risk factor is *alcohol*, because alcohol also plays around with the natural proportions of our night's sleep. You can certainly be more prone to parasomnias after drinking and I advise people who have problems with parasomnias to drink in very careful moderation, if at all. You will realise too perhaps that these risk factors can interact to make things worse – staying up late, drinking, out of your usual routines or trying to deal with stress problems. You get the picture!?

I also want to mention *safety* and what you might call *risk assessment*. If you get out of bed and you are not properly awake, then you are potentially at greater risk of injury. I mentioned before that some sleepwalkers try to go outdoors, even through windows. Some people can be more likely to sleepwalk in unfamiliar places, which of course carries its own risks. It is important therefore that you consider potential risk factors and address these with the family.

Before leaving this section, I want to return briefly to REM parasomnias. Nightmares can often be very challenging to live with and they can be associated with early life trauma or with PTSD. There are effective treatments for nightmare disorder, some are pharmacological and some psychological. There is a technique known as nightmare rescripting, for example, that can help change the nature of the dream content. However, you need professional help with this and with any medication route.

Finally, and still on REM-related events, RBD is most common in middle age or older men. It can occur on its own or it can be associated with motor disorders that occur mainly later on in life, such as Parkinson's disease. It can also be caused or made worse by some medications. So, these are things that should be checked out with your physician. In RBD it is quite common for the bed partner to get injured during the enactment of the sleeper's dreams, and this is the most frequent trigger to help-seeking in my experience. Once again, all the components of management that I have already mentioned are important with RBD, plus a diagnostic PSG assessment if you and your physician feel that this is necessary. There are some drugs that can help reduce or eliminate the symptoms of RBD.

Narcolepsy and hypersomnia

There are a number of key characteristic symptoms associated with *narcolepsy*. Some of these relate to the sleep period and some to daytime. *Hypersomnia* is a term we use for excessive sleepiness and it can occur without all the symptoms of the full narcolepsy syndrome.

During the day, narcolepsy causes extreme daytime sleepiness, and this can present in the form of a *sleep attack*. Normally we fall asleep gradually and we notice the increasing signs of drowsiness along the way. People with narcolepsy too can be aware of their sleepiness, which is very extreme, but they also have sudden sleep attacks that come on more or less out of the blue. Another daytime symptom is called *cataplexy*. This can also occur very suddenly in the form of a cataplectic attack when the body muscles give way, often triggered by extremes of emotion such as humour or anger. During cataplexy however the person remains conscious.

At night, narcolepsy is associated with abnormalities of REM sleep. *Hypnagogic hallucinations* are vivid, dreamlike experiences that occur around sleep-onset, and *hypnopompic hallucinations* are similar phenomena that present in the morning upon wakening. People with narcolepsy go into REM sleep quite readily and so they can experience these transitional dream experiences as if they were part of normal consciousness. There is another unusual symptom known as *sleep paralysis.* This is a period of inability to perform voluntary movements either at sleep-onset or upon awakening. In simple terms the mind wakens up, but the body remains paralysed. So, you will see that narcolepsy is a complex disorder with a number of quite frightening symptoms. You should know however that quite a number of people experience isolated symptoms like sleep paralysis from time to time, and this alone does not indicate narcolepsy.

In recent years, genetic markers for narcolepsy have been identified, and this has improved the accuracy of diagnosis. This can only be fully determined, however, through full PSG assessment, and a procedure known as a *multiple sleep latency test* (MSLT). The MSLT involves attending a sleep laboratory and being given successive 'sleep opportunities' across a period of time. The goal is to detect how rapidly sleep occurs, and to explore the sleep stage characteristics of the sleep that is observed. The possibility of *sleep-onset REM sleep* is one of the features that is being investigated in an MSLT, because this is common in narcolepsy but rare in normal sleepers.

Effective pharmacological treatments have been developed for narcolepsy. These are mostly *stimulant drugs* to help sustain wakeful brain function. Although these drugs are effective, they offer only symptomatic treatment of the presenting problems. *Behavioural factors* such as maintaining a stable sleep pattern, avoiding sleep deprivation, and taking scheduled daytime naps also help. Indeed, despite having this disorder of excessive sleepiness, people with narcolepsy don't always sleep well at night so some cognitive therapeutics from the CBT toolbox can be useful.

How do I get further help?

We started in Part Two with the idea of screening for the possibility that you may have a sleep problem other than insomnia. You have now read this additional chapter to help you to clarify that possibility. So, I hope that you are a bit further on in your own thinking on the matter. If you still think that this may be the case, the next step should be to make an appointment to see your doctor. Take your new-found knowledge, your thoughts and concerns with you to that appointment. You can then discuss the possibility of referral to a specialist sleep clinic if that seems to be the best way forward.

Glossary

actigraph a simple device, usually worn on the wrist, that measures body movement and provides an estimate of time spent awake and time spent asleep.

acute insomnia or transient insomnia is short-term sleep disturbance normally associated with situational or life stressors.

advanced sleep phase syndrome (ASPS) a circadian disorder of sleep where the 'body clock' is set to fall asleep early and to wake early.

alpha rhythm the EEG signal of quiet wakefulness when the eyes are closed.

articulatory suppression a cognitive therapeutic to prevent unimportant mental content from being processed. Articulatory suppression is one form of 'thought-blocking'.

attention bias a tendency to selectively focus, to find your attention drawn to something. In the case of insomnia, the focus is upon sleep and wakefulness.

attention–intention–effort an insomnia process where attention bias leads to intentional sleep and then to effortful sleep, all of which cause wakefulness.

attributions the beliefs that people hold about the causes of a problem.

autogenic training a relaxation therapeutic that emphasises passive relaxation and letting go. Similar to mindfulness.

automaticity the natural and involuntary process of sleep in good sleepers. This is disrupted by attention–intention–effort in insomnia.

baseline the measurement taken as a starting point to describe a problem.

beta activity the EEG signal of alert wakefulness.

body scan a cognitive therapeutic commonly used as part of 'mindfulness'.

case conceptualisation shared understanding of how a problem has developed, what keeps it going, and how best to treat it; also called 'formulation'.

catastrophic thinking spiralling thought processes that are exaggerated, irrational, negative and emotional. Usually addressed using 'cognitive restructuring' or 'paradoxical intention'.

chronic insomnia or persistent insomnia is the complaint of difficulty initiating and/or maintaining sleep that occurs 3 or more nights per week, for at least 3 months, and that is associated with daytime impairment of mood or functioning.

chronotype the particular 'clock type' that is associated with circadian preference.

circadian preference the genetic predisposition that determines when we are most likely to be asleep and awake. For example, 'eveningness' is typical of 'owls' and 'morningness' of 'larks'.

circadian rhythm the regular sleep–wake cycle that is determined by a 'body clock' mechanism in the brain. The circadian system acts as the timer for when sleep occurs.

cognitive control a cognitive therapeutic used in the evening to address thoughts that may interfere with sleep. Also known as 'putting the day to rest'.

cognitive restructuring a cognitive therapeutic useful in 'problem solving'. In simple terms it is rational thinking. Cognitive restructuring is a reappraisal technique used to address 'negative automatic thoughts'.

comorbidity the presence of two or more disorders occurring at the same time. The association between them is not necessarily a causal one.

conditioned arousal the learned association of going to bed, and of attempts to sleep in bed, with wakefulness rather than with successful sleep.

delayed sleep phase syndrome (DSPS) a circadian disorder of sleep where the body clock is set to fall asleep late and to wake late.

Diagnostic and Statistical Manual of Mental Disorders (DSM) a schedule used by mental health professionals to diagnose mental health problems.

differential diagnosis establishing which of two conditions is associated with signs and symptoms that may be similar. 'Comorbidity' is also a possibility.

early morning awakening insomnia that is characterised by being unable to return to sleep following a final awakening that is too early.

electroencephalography (EEG) the measurement of electrical activity in the brain from scalp electrodes.

electromyography (EMG) the measurement of muscle activity using electrodes attached to the body (commonly to the chin and legs).

electro-oculography (EOG) the measurement of eye movements using electrodes attached at the side of the eye sockets.

Five Principles of Good Sleep Health principles that establish an effective pro-sleep mindset based on valuing, prioritising, personalising, trusting and protecting sleep.

formulation shared understanding of how a problem has developed, what keeps it going, and how best to treat it; also called 'case conceptualisation'.

hypersomnia excessive daytime sleepiness, and in the case of depression, excessive sleep duration.

hypervigilant thinking anxious, fearful or panicky thinking, that becomes intense and is often associated with a sense of threat.

hypnogram a graphical presentation of sleep showing transitions between sleep stages in fine detail across the night.

hypnotic dependence psychological and/or physical dependence on a sedative sleep medication. There may be 'rebound insomnia' when the person stops the medication abruptly.

hypnotic drugs prescription medicines that are commonly known as sleeping pills.

imagery training a cognitive therapeutic where practised mental stories can be visualised to focus attention on nice experiences rather than fearful or unpleasant trains of thought.

insomnia disorder the medical term for a clinically important insomnia problem. See 'chronic insomnia'.

International Classification of Diseases a schedule used by health professionals to diagnose medical disorders.

International Classification of Sleep Disorders (ICSD) a schedule used by sleep experts to diagnose different sleep disorders.

melatonin a naturally occurring brain hormone that helps to regulate circadian rhythm.

meta-analysis a scientific study that combines data from a number of 'randomised controlled trials' to establish the level of confidence in a treatment effect.

micro-arousal a brief arousal from sleep lasting a few seconds.

microsleep a lapse into sleep lasting a few seconds. Microsleeps are common when a person is sleep deprived or excessively sleepy, and they can be dangerous e.g. when driving.

mindfulness a cognitive and relaxation therapeutic that emphasises awareness of where you are and what you are doing without overreacting or becoming overwhelmed.

mixed insomnia insomnia that is characterised by difficulties in both getting to sleep and in returning to sleep during the night.

multiple sleep latency test (MSLT) a test of daytime sleepiness that indicates how sleep deprived a person is.

narcolepsy a sleep disorder characterised by excessive sleepiness, sleep attacks, and a number of other specific features.

negative automatic thoughts interpretations of what we think and experience where attention is by default focused on negative factors and consequences.

nightmare disorder vivid and emotional dreams occurring during REM sleep, often recurrent.

night terrors sometimes called sleep terrors. The person experiencing a night terror remains partly asleep but the part of the brain controlling emotion and particularly the fear response is active. Occurs during non-REM sleep.

non-REM sleep sleep stages 1, 2 and 3 form 75 per cent of the night's sleep, with stage 2 being the most common.

obstructive sleep apnoea a sleep-related breathing disorder involving breathing pauses during sleep, and sleep fragmentation, that make people excessively sleepy during the daytime.

off-label prescribing prescription medicines that are recommended treatments for a different condition. For example, pills for other conditions that have sedative side-effects may be prescribed to people with insomnia.

paradoxical insomnia a complaint of insomnia whereby people feel that they hardly ever sleep at all; formerly known as sleep-state misperception.

paradoxical intention a cognitive therapeutic to address sleep preoccupation and sleep effort.

parasomnias a group of sleep disorders characterised by nocturnal activity during partial arousals from sleep or transitions between sleep stages. The most common non-REM parasomnias are sleepwalking, sleeptalking and night terrors. The most common REM parasomnias are nightmares.

periodic limb movement disorder (PLMD) periodic limb movements during sleep involving repetitive jerky movements. They can constitute a disorder when they disrupt sleep. Often associated with 'restless legs syndrome'.

personalised behavioural medicine the selection of the right components of treatment for the individual and applying them in the most effective way.

polysomnography (PSG) the detailed measurement of the sleep process using many (poly) measurements including EEG, EMG and EOG. PSGs are usually conducted in a lab, but there are portable systems for home use.

problem solving a cognitive therapeutic that helps you to see problems as challenges to be solved. It often involves using rational thinking like 'cognitive restructuring'.

progressive relaxation training a relaxation therapeutic that involves systematic muscle tension-release cycles, typically accompanied by breathing control, 'imagery training' and 'autogenic training'.

psychophysiological insomnia insomnia caused largely by psychological factors including conditioned arousal in bed and sleep-related worry. See also 'attention–intention–effort'.

putting the day to rest a cognitive therapeutic used in the evening to address thoughts that may interfere with sleep. Also known as 'cognitive control'.

randomised controlled trial (RCT) a scientific study that tests the effectiveness of a treatment under controlled conditions, taking account of chance and often also of placebo factors.

rapid eye movement sleep (REM sleep) periods of sleep when the body is very still but the brain is very active (often dreaming). Named after its characteristic eye movements.

rebound insomnia an insomnia caused by abrupt withdrawal effects from drugs of a sedative nature, occurring particularly when there is hypnotic dependence.

relapse prevention making preparations mentally and behaviourally for the likelihood that symptoms recur from time to time. Being ready to put CBT quickly into practice to prevent problems getting worse.

REM sleep behaviour disorder a sleep disorder characterised by retained muscle tone during sleep, and the 'acting out' of dream content.

restless legs syndrome (RLS) a sleep disorder characterised by unpleasant sensations in the legs, relieved only by movement. Often associated with 'periodic limb movements'.

sleep compression therapy a behavioural therapeutic that improves 'sleep efficiency' by steadily reducing (compressing) time spent in bed. A graduated form of 'sleep restriction therapy'.

sleep condition indicator (SCI) an assessment tool used to score sleep pattern and sleep quality against diagnostic criteria for insomnia disorder.

sleep deprivation the consequences of insufficient sleep involving fatigue, daytime sleepiness, and increased drive for recovery sleep.

sleep efficiency (SE) the proportion of time in bed that is spent asleep, expressed as a percentage.

sleep effort scale a measure of the attention-intention-effort pathway which quantifies the extent to which trying too hard to sleep has become a problem.

sleep homeostasis the drive for sleep that is governed primarily by the amount of time spent awake. The homeostat tries to create a balance by satisfying sleep needs.

sleep hygiene practices that address lifestyle and bedroom environment factors that are conducive to good sleep.

sleep inertia a temporary state of low arousal immediately after awakening from sleep when it feels like you have not properly woken up.

sleep-maintenance insomnia insomnia that is characterised by waking up and having difficulties in returning to sleep during the night.

sleep-onset insomnia insomnia that is characterised by difficulties in getting to sleep at the start of the night.

sleep–onset latency (SOL) time taken to fall asleep after going to bed and putting out the light.

sleep restriction therapy a behavioural therapeutic that improves 'sleep efficiency' by spending less time in bed.

sleep stages sleep is divided into different stages using standard scoring criteria: non-REM stages 1 to 3 (sometimes called N1, N2 and N3), REM sleep, wake and movement time.

sleep state misperception former term for paradoxical insomnia.

sleepwalking sometimes called somnambulism. The sleepwalker remains partly asleep but the part of the brain controlling body movement is active. Occurs during non-REM sleep.

sleep window the opportunity for sleep that you give yourself, between time of going to bed and time of rising from bed.

social jetlag the difference between the timing of sleep on workdays versus free days (commonly weekends).

stimulus control therapy a behavioural therapeutic that strengthens the bed–sleep connection associated with normal good sleep.

thought-blocking a cognitive therapeutic to prevent unimportant mental content from being processed. Articulatory suppression is one form of 'thought-blocking'.

time in bed (TIB) the period from retiring to rising.

total sleep time (TST) hours and minutes of sleep on a given night.

total wake time (TWT) the total of SOL plus WASO.

transient insomnia or acute insomnia is short-term sleep disturbance normally associated with situational or life stressors.

wake time after sleep-onset (WASO) the total time spent awake during night-time awakenings (after first falling asleep).

zeitgeber or time-giver. Factor that influences when we sleep and when we are awake. The most influential zeitgeber is natural light.

Useful Organisations

The author

<u>Websites</u>
Personal: https://www.colinespie.com

University of Oxford:
  https://www.ndcn.ox.ac.uk/team/colin-espie

<u>Twitter</u>
@ProfEspie

Insomnia and sleep problems

American Academy of Sleep Medicine: https://aasm.org

Asian Sleep Research Society: www.asrsonline.org

Australasian Sleep Association: https://www.sleep.org.au

British Sleep Society: https://www.sleepsociety.org.uk

Canadian Sleep Society: https://css-scs.ca

European Sleep Research Society: https://esrs.eu

National Sleep Foundation: https://www.thensf.org

SBSM:

Sleep Research Society:
    https://www.sleepresearchsociety.org

World Sleep Society: https://worldsleepsociety.org/

Psychotherapies and CBT

Asian Cognitive and Behaviour Therapy Association:
    www.asiancbt.weebly.com

Association for Behavioural and Cognitive Therapies:
    www.abct.org

Australian Association for Cognitive and Behaviour
    Therapy: www.aacbt.org.au

British Association for Behavioural and Cognitive Psycho-
    therapies: https://babcp.com

European Association for Behavioural and Cognitive
    Therapies: www.eabct.eu

International Association for Cognitive Psychotherapy:
    www.the-iacp.com

Latin-American Association of Analysis, Behavioural
    Modification and Cognitive and Behavioural Therapies:
    www.alamoc-web.org

World Confederation of Cognitive and Behavioural
    Therapies: www.wccbt.org

Sleepio

Need more help
with your sleep?
Try Sleepio – the online
sleep improvement
programme developed
by Prof. Colin A. Espie.

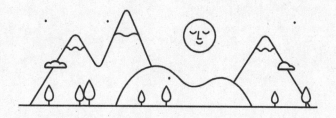

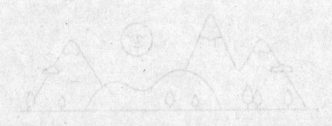

Index

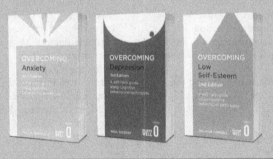